Hug Everyone You Know

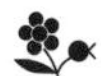

Praise for

Hug Everyone You Know

"*Hug Everyone You Know* is a compelling memoir about the importance of community while navigating a life crisis such as cancer. As an oncology nurse and a cancer survivor myself, I found Martin's writing to be a refreshingly real depiction of life as a cancer patient. Her writing is a testimony to the endurance of the human spirit, the importance of love and community, and the need for hope every day of the journey."

—Story Circle Reviews

"This book will show readers the power of human connectivity and how sharing our experience can become an inspiring journey, not only for those who listen to us, but for us who live it. *Hug Everyone You Know: A Year of Community, Courage, and Cancer* is a painful and empowering journey, a book that will speak to those undergoing any hopeless situation; it's a gift to receive, use and pass on. This book will give readers the strength and the inspiration to name their suffering and to triumph over it. It's exciting, informative and, above all, entertaining." —Readers' Favorite

"This is a great story: inventive, informative, and irresistibly readable. Quite an accomplishment when the subject is cancer. Brava."

—Odette Heideman, Editor, *Epiphany Magazine*

"*Hug Everyone You Know* captures beautifully the terror and anxiety—as well as the awkwardness and occasional humor—that follow a diagnosis of breast cancer, and the salvation to be found in the love and support of family and friends. Peering deeply into the experience through a detailed assessment of her fears, the bonds she shares with others, and hitherto unknown reserves of courage, Martin shares revelatory insights about her willingness to go to any lengths to fight the disease because of what she has learned about the preciousness of life."

—Andrew Botsford, Editor and Visiting Professor, Stony Brook Southampton University

"I picked up this book on a early Sunday afternoon and did not set it down until I was finished. The writing is like being with a long-time friend. It is honest and you can feel the love that the author exudes and surrounds her. Being an escapist, I was reluctant to read a journey on cancer because it hits too close to home. However, quite the opposite is the effect the book had on me. It is not clinical and if you are going through treatments I would imagine you would find it comforting. I would recommend this book to anyone. It is a very enjoyable read."

—Monique Abel, GHT Book Club

"This is an honestly written account of the challenges that face women and families confronting a breast cancer diagnosis. It passionately illustrates the ability of women and their 'Everyones' to find strength."

—Karen Schmitt, MA, BSN Director, Manhattan Cancer Services Program New York Presbyterian/Columbia

"*Hug Everyone You Know* is more than a memoir of combating cancer head on—it is a personal account of the love of family and friends; Antoinette's 'Everyone' who supported her and witnessed her bravery over an arduous year. As Antoinette retells her story, she tries not to give a voice to cancer. Yet, she reveals her innermost thoughts, sharing experiences and fears through the journal she kept during her year of treatment. The author's narrative is carefully woven together with the e-mail exchanges she has with her loved ones. Long after the book is finished, its message continues to linger: life is bigger than itself when fueled by determination and love."

—Janice Gatta, MS/CCC-SLP, Babes Against Cancer Fundraising Committee—Southward Ho Country Club

"I am inspired by Antoinette's courage and spirit. She is blessed—blessed with her husband and children, blessed with her family and friends, and blessed with her doctors and nurses. Being in the medical field, it's a shot of reality seeing it from the patient's point of view, with the day in and day out struggles of life compounded with the diagnosis. This book brought a face to breast cancer and I feel privileged and honored that she shared it with me. I will hug everyone I know, now and forever."

—Barbara M. O'Brien RN, Director of Cancer Services Program of Staten Island Staten Island University Hospital

"Martin has a way of writing that really captured my attention and brought me into her story. I felt like her best friend."

—Kathryn Gates-Ferris, MS, MPA, CHT, Avon Project Director CAI Global

"Filled with fresh air, light, and life, *Hug Everyone You Know* is an intimate conversation with an intelligent, funny survivor. The voice rings true, and the insights resonate well beyond the cancer moment."

—Joni Rodgers, *New York Times* best-selling author of *Bald in the Land of Big Hair*

Hug Everyone You Know

A Year of Community, Courage, and Cancer

Antoinette Truglio Martin

SHE WRITES PRESS

Published 2017
Printed in the United States of America
ISBN: 978-1-63152-262-8 pbk
ISBN: 978-1-63152-263-5 ebk
Library of Congress Control Number: 2017939855

Book design by Stacey Aaronson

For information, address:
She Writes Press
1563 Solano Ave #546
Berkeley, CA 94707

She Writes Press is a division of SparkPoint Studio, LLC.

For my mom, Diana Mastropaolo Truglio,
and my grandmother, Margherita Mastropaolo—the women who inspired fierce perseverance.

For my grandma, Mary Truglio,
who always believed that I was a writer.

contents

Part I: Diagnosis and Detours

Part II: Revelations and Tribulations

Part III: Home Stretch

❊

introduction

Most of us live within a complicated web of relationships. We admire some people with whom we have these relationships for their fortitude. We like others for their humor and interests. We love those whom we are born to, those we birthed, and those who stir the passions in our heart and mind. Our relationship web can be a massive collection of beings, all with unique needs to recognize and gifts to share. We are not alone. We have our *Everyone.*

When a crisis hits—when life throws us a detour—our circles tighten, ready to worry and wanting to help. Everyone feels the pluck on the thread, the change in the force. Nothing is about one; everything is connected.

A breast cancer diagnosis was my detour. It was not planned. It was not expected. As an overly squeamish, wimpy crybaby, just thinking about the series of protocols and treatments I was faced with made me dizzy with nausea.

When this crisis hit, My Everyone felt the shake in the web. The trick, I learned, was to keep the anxiety at bay so that My Everyone, especially those closest to my heart—my daughters, my husband, and my parents—would not be frightened. I could not allow the cancer to be all about me.

For me, the written word has always held a power of expression that I cannot quite articulate. Throughout my remembered life I have filled volumes of composition notebooks, locked diaries, and journals with my deepest thoughts. My ramblings have paced my doubts and placed my anxieties in calm waters, allowing me to see through each crisis and trust in a glass half-full rather than awaiting the end of days. When my biggest life crisis took the form of cancer, I picked out an ugly spiral notebook and let the written word do the ranting, the screaming, the questioning, and the recording. With the help of journaling, I could calm down and face the day—I was able to reach out to My Everyone without panicking anyone, especially myself.

Ultimately, however, I credit the magic of e-mails with saving my sanity. Because of e-mailing, I did not have to explain over and over again the latest episode of cancer treatment; instead, I was able to send a single note to My Everyone. This saved me from hearing and saying the words out loud.

There were of course phone calls and real conversations with my husband, Matt, my mom, my sisters, and my close friends as well. But the e-mails made the initial reporting easy and elicited the support I sought from my wider network.

In writing this memoir, I culled through reams of these e-mails. My aim was to capture the different voices and loving intentions I received from My Everyone. The collections proved that I was never alone. I could count on prayers, positive energies, virtual hugs, and real embraces to keep me focused—hugs, the elixir to panicky anxiety. I learned to be courageous, thanks to My Everyone and the love they wrapped around me.

cast of email contacts

My Relations

My Girls

Sara — My eldest daughter, the artist
Hallie — My middle daughter, most sensitive and sweet
Robyn — My youngest daughter, my adventure baby

My Sisters

Mary — My sister, the second-oldest of the four of us
Barbara — My youngest sister, who lives in faraway Virginia
Heidi — My sister-in-law, Matt's youngest sister

My Cousins

Gloria — One of my many cousins who shared my childhood
Stefano — My Roman cousin who recently immigrated to America

My Friends

Pam B & Nick
Coll & Dan
Chris & Fluke

These friends date back to high school. We formed a cooking group called I-Night some twenty-five years ago, and they all live nearby, allowing us to share vacations, adventures, and lots of laughs.

Irene
My childhood friend, as close to my heart as my sisters

Renee

My college roommate and dear friend

Anne St. John

Another dear friend I've stayed close to through the years

Colleen

The bravest friend I could ever have as we faced cancer together

Dr. Pam
Lisa
Julie

My long-time beach bum pals — we play hard and enjoy our beach adventures season after season

Joi
Addie

Fellow writers I have had the privilege to know and love

Sherry
Janet

Colleagues from the best agency I ever worked for. Sherry is a speech pathologist, and Janet is a physical therapist. They are both breast cancer survivors. Their advice and friendship proved to be so valuable.

part one

Diagnosis and Detours

chapter one

And So It Begins

Wednesday, February 7, 2007

Matt dragged me back to New York University Clinical "C" Center. We took a morning rush-hour train from Ronkonkoma to Penn Station. I wanted to walk the remaining six blocks to quell my anxiety.

It was so much colder this day than it had been the previous week when we ventured into the Clinical "C" Center. That day, the breast surgeon over-kneaded my right breast, unable to feel the deep mass the mammogram had promised. Her sonographer pushed and poked a slippery wand deep into my breast while I struggled to remain still and conscious. When the technician asked me to hum, a gray shadow thickened as the drone reverberated off a rib. A biopsy was ordered for the following week. Ever since, I'd been hoping that this was all a big waste of time for a benign lump.

Frigid winds blew down 34th Street. I wrapped my wool coat tighter and adjusted my hat. Matt held my hand, pulling me behind him, as he weaved through the crowds. The red earflaps on the alpaca hat that Sara, the eldest of our three daughters, had knitted for him danced behind his broad shoulders. Sara worked in Manhattan and planned to meet us for lunch. Matt had the address of a bar with an incredible beer list; we thought it would be a good place to go to celebrate the probable good news after the appointment. I hadn't told Sara the reason for the appointment; I didn't want to worry her, and besides, after a week of thinking myself into it, I believed the lump to be benign.

My anxiety heightened in the waiting room and then even more so in the next room, where they left me to wait once again after having me don a seersucker robe. Thankfully there was plenty of space to pace.

Finally, the doctors arrived, and I was instructed to lie on a hard table. A pathologist, radiologist, nurse, and technician surrounded me. As soon as the poking for the just-right spot started, I faded from consciousness.

I expected this. My squeamish nature has always allowed me to escape discomfort through fainting. I felt my body lighten and fall limp. I could not see but heard distant voices calling my name, debating if they should stop. I mumbled for them just to finish. I passed out again as the pressure mounted and the needle plunged deep into my breast.

Once I was upright, still wrapped in the shapeless robe, I was escorted to a small lab to chat with the pathologist. He asked for my medical history. It was boring. My history was clear of memorable injuries, illnesses, or surgeries. By my thirty-first birthday I had given birth, without anesthesia, to three healthy baby girls. Presently I struggled with blood pressure and weight issues, but I assured the pathologist that I would seriously work on that.

The pathologist reviewed his decades of experience and expertise in studying this insidious disease. Wow, I thought as he rambled, this ancient scientist must have invented the microscope and staining protocols that initially identified pathological cells.

He was giving me way too much of his resumé.

Finally, he came around to the biopsy. Positive. Absolutely positive.

I was speechless. How could this be?

He rattled on as to the depth of the tumor, the size, the need for surgery, and how he admired the skill and manner of my surgeon, Dr. Axelrod. My eyes welled up with tears. I needed to sit down. He patted my shoulder and said, "I will get your mister."

Matt walked into the room, arms laden with coats, hats, and my oversized pocketbook. He took one look at me and said, "Oh, Christ, this doesn't look good."

The pathologist repeated his résumé, the biopsy findings, and the next steps. Matt held my shoulders, let me bury my tears in his chest. He made the appointment with the surgeon while I got dressed.

I could not wait for the elevator. I darted into the stairwell and raced down the stairs and through the glass doors into the street. It was still cold and crowded; all these people were going about their business, unaware that my life had taken a sharp detour.

Matt grabbed my hand as we navigated our way to Penn Station.

"Just get me home," I said.

The early afternoon train was surprisingly crowded. Wedged between a sleeping stranger and Matt, I called Sara as the train pulled out, struggling to keep my voice steady.

"It will be okay, honey. It is small. Not a big deal. I will call you later."

"We can fix this," Matt said for the second time as the train lumbered through the tunnel under the East River.

Matt had always seen problems as engineering projects. He identified a need, came up with a well-planned solution, then executed the solution—and it always worked.

We started dating during the last few months of our high school senior year. Matt was the powerful center on the football team, a boy with thick glasses and an innate talent for understanding and tackling almost any obstacle. I needed a smart friend to help me pass the New York State Physics Regents Exam; he needed a prom date. That was the summer of 1975, and we've been a couple ever since.

During college summer breaks, Matt earned his tuition and expenses by clamming on the Great South Bay. Every summer he kept grumpy motorboat engines running, even if it meant spitting gasoline into sputtering carburetors. In our twenty-seven years of marriage, he had gutted and rebuilt two homes and pieced together small fleets of cars and boats to fit our needs and desires. Matt could fix almost anything. But did he really think he could fix this?

And "we"—he spoke of "we," when it was me who had a growing tumor. Me who had to have the surgery and God knew what else. Me who was suddenly being made to face my mortality. I wanted to cry a sea of tears on that unbearably slow train. This was not supposed to happen. At forty-nine, I had believed that I would skip along into old age with no more than a few bumps and bruises along the way.

In 1985, my second baby, Hallie, was due to be born when Hurricane Gloria ravaged Long Island, leaving us without electric power for a week. Even the hospital had to rely on generators. Luckily, Hallie arrived a week overdue, ten pounds of perfect beauty. That same week, Halley's Comet passed by this hemisphere—but between caring for a hungry infant and her busy two-and-a-half-year-old sister, Sara, and cleaning up from the hurricane's path, I missed it.

When that happened, I vowed, in my robust state of twenty-eight-year-old health, that I would have a birthday bash at 103 to celebrate a fulfilled life and the return of Halley's Comet. For twenty years I had been inviting everyone that came into my life to that party. The women in my mother's family were fierce and lived close to their centurion birthdate. I figured the odds that I would make it to that party in decent mental and physical health, to see the comet's next sweep past Earth, were pretty good.

But today, thoughts of being dependent and possibly facing a shortened life expectancy crowded the train car. I wanted to scream! This could not be happening to me—not now, not ever. I could never be strong enough. I had always believed that God didn't give us tasks we weren't strong enough to endure. I had always been the wimp. I cried. I trembled. I became a large blubbery puddle in the face of the slightest medical challenge.

On top of that, this was such rotten timing! The house was for sale. Our empty nest in Remsenburg, a tidy hamlet on the south shore of Long Island, had been stripped of all its homey comforts, the better to entice picky buyers in a housing bubble crisis. Three different realtors' "For Sale" signs had adorned our front yard for over a year. We had already bought a lot in Sayville, our hometown, twenty-five miles west of Remsenburg, so we could be closer to family and old friends. I was also waiting to be called for an interview to fill a speech therapy vacancy at a school district. Will the call come while I am recovering from surgery, or worse, dealing with treatment side effects? I wondered. Hallie was graduating from SUNY New Paltz in May. Could I postpone any debilitating treatments to see her walk?

I had to call Mom and my sisters. How was I supposed to tell my Hallie and Robyn? I hadn't even told them about the biopsy because it was not supposed to be positive! I could not keep them in coddled ignorance. And what if I could not work? Could we manage with me on disability? And what about the daily housekeeping? Matt could cook and take care of basic upkeep, but he would find any excuse—work responsibilities, promising fishing reports, and/or boat maintenance—to not have to vacuum or do dishes.

These thoughts and more rambled through my head as I pressed quiet tears into Matt's coat. The sleeping stranger on my other side stirred and shrugged his head into the window frame. Matt kept squeezing my hand, promising that it would all be okay.

As the train rumbled on, I suddenly realized I would need my husband more in the months to come than I had ever needed anyone. If I had to depend on one thing, I could depend on him to remain steady and calm. He would not be a chest-beating martyr or an emotionally detached ghost. He would be a rock. Each hand squeeze assured me that this was the truth.

Damn it, the biopsy was positive! I have cancer. How am I supposed to do this?

chapter two

The Telling

I called my sister Mary as the train was slowing toward Jamaica Station. She had left me several messages voicing her suspicion that something had gone wrong. She was the director of the Women's Outreach Network, a mobile mammography program, and had been instrumental in getting me my initial appointment with the breast surgeon.

"Oh my God, Ann!" she gasped when I gave her the news. "I can't believe this is happening to you. I mean, nine times out of ten, my patients go in for a biopsy, and it is nothing!"

"The pathologist said it's small and seems to be contained." I was kind of lying; I had no real memory of what the pathologist said. Matt grumbled, reminding me to keep my voice down. The slumbering neighbor sighed into his scarf.

"Well, that is good news. I can send you some websites that are very helpful, and there are blogs, too," Mary said. "It's important to educate yourself before you agree to anything. There is—"

"Mary, I've got to go. I'm on the train and have to call Mom. I can't talk now." I wasn't ready to listen to Mary's take-charge voice. I am her elder by sixteen months, but she's always been the bossypants with all the answers.

Dad answered on the first ring.

"No! No! Like your mother, only you are so much younger!" He sobbed as he passed the phone to Mom.

She peppered me with questions. I repeated my version of the pathologist's findings: positive, small, probably nothing else involved, all good news considering the diagnosis.

"This could be no more than a small incision. The mass gets sucked out, a Band-Aid is put on, and that can be that." I was making this up. I should have used the line with Dad, who grabbed on to any best-case scenario in a crisis. Mom was not convinced.

My mother, a retired high school biology teacher, a breast cancer survivor, and the founder of Women Outreach Network knew all the statistics, procedures, and outcomes concerning breast cancer. I could not distract her with my rambling imagination.

"Listen, Antoinette, you just have to do what you are told. It is not a death sentence." Her voice crumbled as she took a breath. "No matter what, you have to buck up and just get through this."

She was referring to my aversion to invasive procedures—for anyone's body, but especially mine. The sight of deep wounds, stitches, and the threat of a vein puncturing for a blood test made me lightheaded. I had been fortunate to get through childhood without any bloody accidents. While studying anatomy in college, I could not look at the gory details of the photographs. The line illustrations were good enough for me to memorize origins and insertions. Thankfully, whenever my daughters or our fearless dog, Petie, had gotten a nasty gash over the years, there had always been someone else nearby who could assess the situation, administer first aid, and drive to the emergency room. The most I could ever do was to hold a towel over the laceration and look the other way.

I promised my mother that I would speak to her later and hung up the phone. The two calls had exhausted me. Winter dusk was already darkening the western sky. The train parking lot lights glowed. I turned off my phone. I could not repeat everything again. Since Mary had the news, everyone in the Western Hemisphere was now in the know. The home answering machine would be flashing.

I did not want to go home. Matt realized we had not eaten since the egg-white omelets and coffee we'd had for breakfast.

"Let's get a drink and dinner at the Cull House," he suggested. "I'm starving."

The Cull House had been our favorite watering hole when we lived in Sayville. The rugged cottage near the busy boatyards and Fire Island ferry terminals had remained in business as other, more upscale Main Street restaurants turned over every few years. The local gem's comfort seafood fare and familiar staff had kept the place humming for over twenty years. Even when we moved to Remsenburg, Matt and I had continued to drop in at the Cull House on a regular basis to meet friends and enjoy a satisfying meal.

The restaurant was quiet, as expected on an early mid-week evening. During the summer, the place was hopping, with the indoor and outdoor tables full and all the bar stools occupied. But on this winter night, only one other table was taken.

Mike, the bartender, waved for us to take any seat in the dining room. The waitress brought us our usual: Matt's Tanqueray martini, straight up with olives, and a gin and tonic for me.

I pretended to browse the specials. "I don't think I can eat," I mumbled.

"I'll have a cup of chowder, and we'll share a fried fisherman's platter," said Matt to the waitress. When she walked away, he held my hands across the table and smiled.

"Maybe this is all a mistake," I said. "This is not supposed to happen."

We walked into our house before six o'clock that night. Petie, our Jack Russell Terrier, greeted us and implored someone to take him outside. While Matt walked him, I re-rehearsed what I was going to say to my daughters. This was going to be incredibly difficult. First, I had to call Sara back. Now twenty-four, she was a graduate of the Pratt Institute and had been working as product photographer by day and freelance artist at night. She lived in a tight railroad flat on a narrow street in Greenpoint, Brooklyn. It was a trendy neighborhood with a pierogi deli and upscale markets on the corners.

No answer. I left her a message to call me.

Next I punched in Hallie's number.

She picked up on the first ring. "What's up?"

"Hi, honey, how are you?"

"Exhausted! I've got this big paper due and it's freezing in the apartment, and I have to get to the newspaper tonight to look over the copy."

I gave her a quick version of my day. She immediately cried, interjecting *Oh no-s!* and *It can't be*-s*!*. Hallie had always been sensitive, quick with tears and grief. I answered her questions as cheerfully as possible.

"Should I come home, Mom? Can I see you?" she sobbed.

"No! I do not want you home. I don't need anyone disrupting their schedules now. What you can do for me is be well and do well in school. This is your last semester, Hallie. Don't blow it!" I took a breath. I had to watch my temper with her. She was easily offended and was bound to cry another volley of tears. What I really wanted to do was crawl through the telephone line, hug her tight, and have a good cry with her. She and I were so much alike: big and tough on the outside, marshmallows on the inside.

Matt answered his cell phone. It was Sara. While I said my good-byes to Hallie, he spoke to our eldest daughter. She asked questions; he answered truthfully. He knew he didn't need to sugarcoat things for Sara.

Before I hung up with Hallie, Matt and I traded phones. I repeated Matt's answers to Sara while Matt spoke softly to Hallie. Before Sara hung up, she said she would probably call back later with more questions. Hallie hung up with the promise to make herself a cup of tea and meet her friends at the college newspaper to finish the next day's copy.

Now we had to call Robyn. Brooklyn and New Paltz were a few hours' drive from one another, but Robyn had chosen to go to Fredonia, the most western SUNY campus in New

York State. Impulsively jumping into the car for a weekend in Fredonia would never happen. Although Robyn had made friends and liked the freedom of the college experience during her freshman fall semester, she continued to question if college was right for her. I'd lectured her that a young woman in today's world needed letters after her name to prove she could do and finish something and be qualified to do so much more—so, resigned, she'd left for Fredonia just a few weeks earlier for the spring semester.

Matt broke down and cried into a paper towel. "Our baby is going to have the hardest time understanding all this."

"I have to call her before Sara or Hallie—or Mary—do," I said. "It would be better if she heard from me first."

Robyn was not a crier, nor one to ask questions. She listened and occasionally interjected an "Are you sure?" She, too, asked if I wanted her home. I told her to stay put for now. We could talk any time.

Over the next few hours, each one of my girls called back at least twice. Hallie, by the second call, was calm. I confirmed that we were still going to her outdoor roller derby exhibition in a few weeks. Sara wanted to hear everything repeated. Robyn called to ask what a lumpectomy was and called back an hour later to say good night. Relieved that they all sounded calm, I decided to send them an e-mail.

From: Mommy
To: Sara, Hallie, & Robyn
Date: Wednesday, February 7, 2007 at 10:43 p.m.
Subject: Reassurance

Girls, I am so happy I got to speak to each of you tonight. Yes, this is a shock. I honestly went into the biopsy believing it was nothing, that I had dodged a bullet. The good news is that this is NOT, I repeat, NOT a death sentence. It really should be a few months of disruption. The site is very small, and there does not seem to be anything else involved. So, what I need for you girls to do is to keep focused, keep in touch, and most importantly, keep calm. I need to trust that you will be OK with the news I share with you. Without the drama, I can keep you in the loop. I am very lucky to have your daddy as my rock (as he has always been). I just need you girls to be strong too. We will get through this a little wiser. As far as I am concerned, we are still selling the house, building a new home, and figuring out a way to buy a beach house. I am waiting for a call from Remsenburg-Speonk schools for a job interview. I have been waiting for this call for thirteen years. Wouldn't it be funny if I get the job and we move twenty-five miles away?! There is a lot to do, so much to look forward to and work towards.

Good night, my girls. We will talk soon. Talk to each other, talk to Dad, talk to me. This will all be over and done with soon. Love you all so much.

Mommy

From: Hallie
To: Mommy
Date: Wednesday, February 7, 2007 at 10:51 p.m.
Subject: Reassurance

I love you, too, Mommy. We'll be OK, promise.

~

From: Robyn
To: Mom
Date: Wednesday, February 7, 2007 at 11:23 p.m.
Subject: Reassurance

Love you, Mom!

~

From: Sara
To: Mom
Date: Thursday, February 8, 2007 at 12:23 a.m.
Subject: Friday

I was thinking of coming home on Friday night for dinner. I have to go back on Saturday, but I just feel like coming home for a night.

~

From: Mom
To: Sara
Date: Thursday, February 8, 2007 at 12:44 a.m.
Subject: Friday

When on Friday? If you get to Ronkonkoma by 4:30/5:00, I can pick you up. What would you like for dinner?

From: Sara

To: Mom

Date: Thursday, February 8, 2007 at 3:03 a.m.

Subject:Friday

I can't leave work until 5, so I could probably get into Speonk by 8:30. I don't know what I want for dinner—no mango salsa on fish!

chapter three

Technology Solutions

The phone was problematic. I cringed every time I said or heard the words *biopsy, cancer,* and *tumor.* It was grueling being cheerful while the reality of my situation bore down on my fragile calm. But I had sisters, my mother, and close friends to inform. I needed them.

Over the previous few years, I had used e-mail as my preferred mode for quick communications. I had never been very chatty on the phone, even with my closest friends. E-mail allowed me to keep close with people whom I could not see on a regular basis. It allowed me to send quick messages, letters of encouragement, and carefully crafted words of advice and gratitude so much more thoughtfully than I ever could in my stumbling dialogue. I quickly realized that this was another time when e-mail would most likely serve me best.

So, that first night, I stayed up late (sleep was evading me anyway) to write a light e-mail to my sisters. What a relief to type the words without listening to them!

From: Antoinette
To: Barbara, Irene
Date: Thursday, February 8, 2007 at 3:52 a.m.
Subject: FYI

I am sorry, but I cannot make any more phone calls. I am sure that you have already heard through the rapid-fire grapevine that a biopsy I had was positive. So I am on a journey I didn't sign up for. The good news is that it is small, and I am in good hands at the NYU Clinical "C" Center. I think this will be a nuisance—a bump in the road more than anything else. I'm OK, Matt is OK. The girls were told (worst part), and Mom and Dad are OK too. So, right now, we are OK. I will keep you in the loop. Take care of yourselves.

Hug everyone you know.
Ann

From: Barbara
To: Antoinette
Date: Thursday, February 8, 2007 at 12:03 p.m.
Subject: FYI

You are right—this is an annoyance, not a catastrophe! While you are under the knife, do you want anything tucked? (he-hehe) OK, stress makes this stuff so much worse, so plenty of time in the hot tub and being pampered is prescribed. Kisses!

Barbara

From: Irene
To: Antoinette
Date: Thursday, February 8, 2007 at 7:01 p.m.
Subject: FYI

Yes, Mary did call last night. In talking with my cancer patients, it seems that the waiting is the hardest part. Imagination is a powerful thing. But with the size of the mass and your rapid access to the right MDs, it sounds like your description, a bump in the road, is perfect.

I am sure telling the girls was the most difficult thing to do. Running home is probably the first thing they wanted to do. I hope they are OK. Thank you for keeping me posted. Your phone must be ringing off the hook with information seekers. E-mail works for me. Let me know when the surgery is scheduled. Lots of LOVE and positive thoughts.

Irene
P.S. I hope you are journaling the journey you did not sign up for.

~

Journaling the journey? My sisters knew that I scribbled in pretty covered notebooks. From my earliest memory, I had always said, "I want to be a writer when I grow up." But a practical life robbed me of the time and energy necessary to be a true writer. I'd had a few essays published and wrote regular columns for a couple of local papers. My proudest writing accomplishment thus far had been a children's book, *Famous Seaweed Soup.* What a thrill to see my story illustrated so beautifully, bound and sitting on library shelves and children's laps. As incredible as it was, I soon learned that one cannot quit the day job after writing one children's book. My other children's stories languished in a box, filed alongside stacks of rejection letters. I let writing become a hobby rather than the calling it began as—one that grew dimmer as grown-up responsibilities mounted. But journaling remained a constant in my life. I aimed to write daily but typically managed to do so only sporadically.

Irene was right. I should journal this journey I did not sign up for. It could be a way to navigate through this nightmare without having to say the words out loud.

Cancer did not deserve a pretty notebook with a ribbon to mark my place. I dug a cheap spiral notebook out of a drawer. *Perfect.* I would dog-ear the pages to mark my place. Here I could rant, ramble, recount, list questions, and scribble notes. Hopefully, writing in this journal would relieve all the chatter in my head and keep cancer out of earshot.

chapter four

The Waiting

My girls called several times during the next few days. This was unusual for us. Typically, our telephone conversations consisted of care package or money requests, and weekly catch-ups. We saved the long conversations for the kitchen counter.

At the office, I kept insanely busy coordinating therapists, updating reports, and visiting families on my early-intervention caseload. I liked most of the families in my charge. The moms typically welcomed me and aired their concerns about their special needs babies with honesty. The visits were aimed to alleviate their fears so that they could take an active part in the therapies their children needed and learn to be effective advocates for their child. There was no better feeling than to see a family relax and enjoy each other.

Working for an agency that relied on staying in the good graces of the county's bottom line, however, was problematic for me. I had been with this agency for a year; I'd spent twenty-five years before that working as a speech/language and/or special education therapist with special needs infants and toddlers, advocating for their needs. I had become very skilled in quickly assessing a situation and rationalizing focused therapy services. The policies for this agency's early intervention coordinators made it difficult to approve intensive therapy services. I frequently had to bite my tongue and keep my recommendations to a minimum.

I leaked the news of my upcoming appointments and surgery to my supervisor and cubicle mates. The women I worked with were understanding and respected the need-to-know code of silence I requested of them. That done, I immersed myself in the mountain of paperwork on my desk, letting everyone else's problems look bigger than mine.

Since I had been relatively successful in communicating the news of my diagnosis—and reassurance that I would be okay—to my daughters and sisters, I decided to e-mail my good friends.

~

From: Antoinette
To: Pam B, Nick, Flaherty Clan, Coll & Dan
Date: Thursday, February 8, 2007 at 2:10 p.m.
Subject: Stuff

Remember that conversation we had last weekend on mammograms and sonograms, and that I had something suspicious enough to have to see a breast surgeon and that she had recommended a biopsy? The biopsy was positive. A surgery date and some kind of treatment protocol will be determined next week. The good news is that the site is very small—very, very small—and there should not be lymph nodes involved, so I am thinking this is going to be a nuisance for a few months. Matt has been great, but I think, well, know, he is going to need his pals to call: man bonding stuff. I'm OK. I think I am more in shock than anything else. I honestly thought I had dodged this bullet.

I was pretty much out cold for the biopsy. Who came up with the idea that biopsies are easy? We'll be in touch. Kisses to all. Hug everyone you know.

Ann

~

From: Pam B
To: Antoinette
Date: Thursday, February 8, 2007 at 2:37 p.m.
Subject: Stuff

YIKES! Not good news. But I am proud of you with the needles. Hang in there, buddy. My love and positive thoughts are coming your way.

Pam

~

From: Dan & Coll
To: Antoinette
Date: Friday, February 9, 2007 at 7:43p.m.
Subject: Stuff

What a shock! What can we do?

Friday, February 9, 2007

Sara rode the train home tonight. She just about flew into my arms. We hugged, rocked, and wiped away our tears in the station parking lot.

"You look good, Ma," she said. Sara wanted to see that I looked the same. Amazing to think that learning a diagnosis can shine a whole different light on one's appearance. I've never felt sick. A person with heart disease, a damaged knee, or a simmering ulcer would have symptoms beyond the regular aches and pains—breathless fatigue, a painful limp, heartburn, something that would call for attention and action. But cancer had slipped in without any warning or invitation.

My mother and grandmother were diagnosed with breast cancer in their post-menopausal years. I had been getting yearly mammograms since my fortieth birthday, yet I never worried. My weight was more of a problem, causing blood pressure and cholesterol issues. I was at my heaviest ever, 230 pounds—Matt's svelte wedding weight some twenty-seven years earlier.

Matt cooked the three of us a delicious dinner: striped bass in a lemon-wine sauce and roasted root vegetables. We shared a bottle of wine. We talked about selling the house; Petie, who had a worrisome heart condition; and the glacial weather. We talked well past midnight with glasses of wine in our hands.

Matt drove Sara to the train station Saturday morning. Before she left, we hugged each other tight, whispering, "I love you" to each other.

"You're one tough mom," she said as she slid into the minivan.

"I have to be," I replied, not really believing my own words.

Matt spent the rest of Saturday in the office, catching up on missed work. I busied myself with cleaning the house, again, in case the realtor found a customer willing to see a house in the throes of winter. I found myself quietly crying as I wiped down the bathroom mirror wall. I kept a wet hand towel around my neck for easy eye and nose wipe access.

Petie followed me through the house hoping I would take the tennis ball in his mouth as a hint. To Petie, a throw-and-fetch game could cure anything.

He finally won. I bundled up, slipped his rainbow sweater over his sinewy body, and took him out to the barren backyard, where I threw the ball for him again and again. Each time, Petie leapt up and caught it on the first bounce. He was a sweet little dog with twenty pounds of solid muscle that constantly twitched to jump and run. He did not realize his oversized heart was interfering with his focused mission to play.

Within fifteen minutes, the cold and Petie's coughing made me call the game. We came in smiling and curled up under a blanket on the couch for a nap. The realtor did not call.

On Sunday, Matt and his pals launched an iceboat in Bellport, a small hamlet on the Great South Bay between Remsenburg and Sayville.

I unsuccessfully fought to don my old skates for the occasion. With the double layer of thick socks I insisted upon wearing to combat the frigid February weather, they were too tight. I gave up, telling myself that the steady northeasterly winds had created so many bumps and fissures in the ice that all my amateur attempts at figure eights and spins would be foiled anyway.

But Matt was committed to sailing on the frozen bay, so I went along to spectate.

I had gone on rides, but on this day, the wind was especially wild. Matt and the other men zipped along on small Great South Bay Scooters, iceboats that were used for winter transportation and sport in the early twentieth century. The metal angle irons on the bottom of these skiffs skated on the ice. A mainsail caught the wind propelling the boat. The shifting of body weight and slight tweaking of the handheld jib kind of steered the vessel. A scooter held an exhilarated crew of three skidding on the ice at a breathtaking rate, bouncing and crunching over the bumps and frozen waves with barely any control to an estimated destination.

There were more than a dozen scooters and one-man iceboats skidding on the ice. I watched the freestyle ballet while sliding on my boots and chatting with fellow onlookers—but within an hour, the cold became too much to bear. I decided to visit my friend Pam, who was recovering from a broken foot.

Pam's home was cozy and warm, with overstuffed chairs and a gas fireplace she was able to adjust with a remote control. I was intrigued and claimed I would have to insist on getting one for my new house, if a new house should ever happen. Over a glass of wine, I reviewed my biopsy and upcoming surgery. Pam listened patiently and agreed that this should be a very short journey. She revealed that our friend Colleen had also had a suspicious scan and was scheduled to see her mother's oncologist. I could only shake my head.

"I have a mammo, sonogram, and bone density test scheduled next week," Pam said.

"Don't skip it," I advised.

I met Matt at my parents' house in Sayville—the big colonial overlooking the Great South Bay that I grew up in—for Sunday dinner. My love of sailing and the sea stem from this house. The bedroom I shared with Mary overlooked the bay, and from our window we witnessed pink sunrises, angry seas crashing into the bulkhead, and nights with shimmering reflections of moonlight.

Sunday dinner was a regular tradition founded in the roots of my Italian heritage. Both of my parents grew up in Brooklyn in similar Italian neighborhoods with extended families living in the same building or within walking distance of each other. My dad's family had a "country house" shared by multiple families in the American Venice area of

Lindenhurst village on Long Island. As a young boy, my dad established his love of fishing and boating and was driven as a young man to continue this lifestyle for his own family. After their marriage in 1956, my parents emigrated from Brooklyn to the suburbs on Long Island.

The exodus back to Brooklyn for Sunday dinner was an unspoken mandatory tradition throughout my childhood. My parents packed the station wagon with their growing clan—myself, my three younger sisters, and my baby brother—in the morning, and after attending Sunday mass, we, along with our aunts, uncles, and cousins, converged at Grandma's second-floor flat. The stairwell was always warm. It smelled like Grandma's house with the aromas of garlic and tomato sauce.

Sunday dinner started in the afternoon and ended sometime before the children needed to go home. Sunday was, after all, a school night. The afternoon and early evening consisted of eating, catching up on family gossip, playing cards, and singing old songs. My cousins, sisters, and I played ball in the street and chased each other through the flat, up and down the stairs, and into the alley. Each one of our names was called from the second-floor window when it was time to come to the table.

Even when Grandma sold her Brooklyn home and moved to Sayville to be closer to her children, grandchildren, and great-grandchildren (her "bonus," as she would say), she held court during the weekly Sunday dinners.

As time passed, some traditions faded away, and others left kicking and screaming, trailing a wake of guilt. Sunday dinner evolved into my parents hosting anyone who would come around every other week or so. Oven-ready mini pizzas, chicken wings, olives, and cheese plates were offered before sitting down to too much macaroni, meaty sauce, and roasted artichokes. Whenever any of my parents' grandchildren entered the house, they would exclaim, "It smells like Sunday at Grandma's!" My mom would reward the complimenting child with a meatball on a fork.

Everyone brought something to add to the gluttony. Since I had gone on the ice earlier on this Sunday, I did not cook my usual eggplant caponata or stuffed sausage bread. Instead, I picked up freshly filled cannoli at the Italian bakery.

I usually enjoyed these Sundays. It gave me and my sisters a chance to catch up with our kids. Plus most of us were in the education field so we always had the latest trend to complain about. Today, though, my cancer diagnosis took center stage. I gave everyone a very brief version of the biopsy episode—I was still having trouble saying the words out loud without stifling a sob. Mom and Mary filled us all in on the latest information on the surgeon and the treatment options, which they intimately knew through their work with the mobile mammography van. My treatment options, they said, were all dependent upon the results of the lumpectomy. They worried about my relatively young age and the fact that I had no pre-menopausal symptoms. Mom had her journey to recount. My sister Diana and sister-in-law Rose told of neighbors, friends, coworkers who had gone through a variety of breast cancer scenarios. A few had not made it through.

Eventually, the topic turned to my sisters' theories on how I would react to treatments. They retold stories from our childhood—various versions of me crying when someone got hurt and there was a lot of blood. There was the time I fainted upon seeing a fresh row of stitches on a cousin's leg. Mom even added a story about the time when the neighbor ran over upon hearing me scream only to discover my mother wrestling a brush through my curls.

I knew they were just trying to lighten the mood with the stories, but it wasn't fun for me. I left the kitchen to sit with Dad, Matt, and my brothers-in-law watching Super Bowl highlights. Silently, I brooded. Although it was true that I was the one who always cried in response to anyone's discomfort and fainted at just the thought of a needle, I decided to keep the details of the upcoming ordeal from my sisters and mom. They were just as scared as I was.

chapter five

Breast Cancer 101

As much as I wanted to know what to expect, I didn't want to know everything. I continued to repeat the mantra, "This is not happening." The appointment with my surgeon was coming up, however, so I decided I should at least understand the lingo. I began to do some research.

Ductal carcinoma is the most common kind of breast cancer. It begins in the lining of the breast ducts. Ductal carcinoma in situ (DCIS) is diagnosed when the cancer cells are only in the lining of the milk ducts and have not spread to other tissues in the breast. If the cancer cells have broken through the ducts and spread to other parts of the breast tissue, it is called invasive ductal carcinoma. Those invasive cancer cells can also spread to other regions of the body.

Lobular carcinoma begins in the lobules of the breast. Lobules are the glands that produce the milk. The cancer cells are found only in the breast lobules in lobular carcinoma in situ, or LCIS. When lobular carcinoma spreads from the lobules to nearby breast tissues, it is called invasive lobular carcinoma and can also spread to other parts of the body. (Are you seeing a pattern here?)

Staging breast cancer is used as part of the diagnosis. It is based on a scale of zero through four. Stage 0 describes non-invasive cancers that remain within their original location. The scale progresses to Stage IV when invasive cancers have spread outside the breast to other parts of the body.

Then there is the estrogen factor. Most breast cancers are estrogen receptors, meaning that they feed on estrogen. I learned that estrogen loves to settle into fat. *Great.* I certainly had plenty of fuel to feed the cancer.

Another possible culprit is the HER2 (human epidermal growth factor receptor-2) gene. The HER2 gene makes HER2 proteins that are breast cell receptors. Normally, HER2 receptors help control how a healthy breast cell grows, divides, and repairs itself. If the HER2 gene is overactive, however, it may cause wild divisions of cells, which can cause the cancer.

Based on this short, self-administered course, I aimed for a very small Stage 0, DCIS estrogen receptor, HER2-negative tumor with negative margins and node involvement. Mostly, I wished for this to be a huge mistake.

chapter six

More Waiting

Tuesday, February 13, 2007

We rode the train to the NYU Clinical Cancer Center. I insisted on walking from Penn Station despite the gray and bitter cold. Anticipating a long wait, I'd packed a tote bag with reports to review, a book, and a few granola bars. Matt had shoved in the morning newspaper before we drove off to the train station.

I had been investigating all kinds of possible scenarios and learning my new language, but I wasn't talking to Matt about them. Although I wanted to understand the terms and options, I did not want to speak the words. Every time I had to say a cancer-related word, anxiety choked my neck, blocking fluency and breath.

I remembered feeling this when Mom went through her treatments eight years earlier. At sixty-six, she'd gone through a biopsy, lumpectomy, chemotherapy, and radiation therapy. She was selected for a new chemo cocktail, complete with a trial of an anti-nausea medication. Although she did not lose her hair, it did turn brittle from the treatments, and she had to eventually cut her mid-back-length tresses short. Her fingernails constantly ripped, and she was uncharacteristically exhausted. Her biggest lament was that she had to reduce her wine consumption. I would call or visit to see how she was doing only to get abbreviated details and assurances.

Mom was a lot braver than I could ever be. She'd even insisted on going to chemotherapy and radiation by herself. She did not want to worry Dad—who, though he always stood strong, was in reality very sensitive when there was distress he could not fix.

As expected, the delay in Dr. Axelrod's waiting room drew close to two hours. Although I'd come prepared with reports and books, I found myself people watching. This whole breast health business was a family affair. Women of all ages, sizes, and religious garb milled in and out of the back rooms. Very few women sat alone. Some women, like me, sat quietly with their men. Others sat with daughters and sons who kept close to their sides, exchanging whispers.

I was drawn to a seemingly young woman with a woolen skullcap pulled close to missing eyebrows. She was tiny, with tight skin covering pronounced cheekbones and a pointed chin. Her muddy eyes, stripped of eyelashes, appeared sunken into a fragile face. She was wrapped in layers of scarves and sweaters and wedged between a man and woman—her parents, I assumed. They each held her bony hands and stared at the wall art in front of them. The girl bobbed her head between the shoulders of her zombie parents.

I could not fathom the anguish this family must be facing.

There could not be any worse pain than experiencing your child's horrid illness and imminent death.

Matt and I had to wait another thirty minutes in Dr. Axelrod's office before finally being seen, which gave me time to browse the photographs and read the licenses and certifications cluttering the walls. A poster-sized book cover with Dr. Axelrod and Rosie O'Donnell's picture on it hung on one wall. Apparently the two had coauthored the book *Bosom Buddies: Lessons and Laughter on Breast Health and Cancer.* A photograph of Hillary Clinton, in her signature First Lady headband, shaking Dr. Axelrod's hand sat on the desk next to family pictures.

Mary had mentioned that Dr. Axelrod was a bit of a celebrity. Despite her notoriety and hectic schedule, she was quick to participate in Women's Outreach Network fundraisers and offer guidance to their cause. "She is the most approachable surgeon with talent in New York City," Mary said.

I was still looking at the Hillary photo when Dr. Axelrod entered the office and patted my folder. "How are you?" she asked.

"I just want to get this over with."

"And we will, and you will be just fine." She looked straight at me with a warm smile. I suddenly felt safe.

Dr. Axelrod began the discussion. She described the schedule of the surgery day and the purpose of each procedure. Between each detail, she was careful to ask both Matt and me if we had any questions. She explained that I would begin the day downtown at St. Vincent's Hospital on West 12th Street with a nuclear radiologist—someone she trusted wholly—who would insert a radioactive dye that would light up the sentinel lymph nodes under my arm. The glow made it easy to find and remove the nodes. A car service would then pick me up and bring me to the NYU Cancer Center, where a radiologist would use a sonogram to insert a wire through my breast to the tumor. This, again, would give her a path directly to the mass, saving a lot of digging around. Then it would be back in the car, whisked to ambulatory surgery at NYU Hospital, two blocks away. There, the lumpectomy would be completed. I should go home that afternoon. We would be given preliminary pathology findings that day. A full report should be completed by the follow-up visit the next week. I would probably need a course of radiation therapy, but definite treatment options would be discussed once we knew what type of cancer was living in my body.

Dr. Axelrod talked about margins, the importance of the lymph node involvement, and how I should heal with little more than a scar on my breast and under my arm. I needed to get an oncologist on board. She had several excellent doctors to refer me to at NYU but encouraged us to explore doctors on Long Island as well.

Dr. Axelrod admitted that the driving around the city just to prepare for surgery seemed daunting, but said that her method had yielded excellent results with minimal damage to the breast and very low incidence of lymphedema, a condition in which excess fluid collected in the arm tissue and caused swelling. She spent the better part of an hour explaining, answering questions, and patiently repeating explanations. When we were through, a smiling nurse entered the office with a pile of paperwork to review. Dr. Axelrod left us with a hearty handshake. She was running late.

Once the paperwork was complete, the nurse asked if we could stay for just another moment. Twenty minutes later, Dr. Axelrod breezed back into her office. She asked if we had any other questions, reassured me that I would be just fine, and said to call if any questions should come up. Before leaving, she gave each of us a hug.

She was worth the wait. I was in excellent hands.

~

From: Antoinette
To: My Everyone
Date: Thursday, February 15, 2007 at 8:41 p.m.
Subject: Update

I am scheduled for surgery: lumpectomy and lymph node dissection on Monday, 2/26. Matt and I will stay in the city for two nights (Sunday and Monday) mostly because there is a lot of prep early on Monday morning. Even though I will be discharged on the same day, it would be better to be in a cozy nearby hotel instead of traveling home for two hours. Matt is thinking of "just in case" scenarios. We will take our time coming home on Tuesday. I plan to be back at work on Thursday. Radiation therapy is most probable; anything else will be recommended once a full report is complete. This should not be too bad—a good scare and nuisance.

Thank you all for your thoughts, good wishes, and support. I will be fine. I'll keep you posted.

Hug everyone you know.
Ann

From: Barbara
To: Antoinette
Date: Thursday, February 15, 2007 at 9:23 p.m.
Subject: Update

OK, Ann, I am sending love, kisses, and happy thoughts. Stress is bad, so happy thoughts.

Barbara

From: Renee
To: Antoinette
Date: Friday, February 16, 2007 at 10:48 a.m.
Subject: Update

You sound like my spunky roommate. Good! And good, too, that you are staying overnight with Matt in a hotel. A great idea to buffer the surgery and work. Do what you have to do to get rid of the "nuisance" and do stuff that's good for you just because you want to. Sending hugs. We'll talk soon.

Renee

From: Colleen
To: Antoinette
Date: Friday, February 16, 2007 at 3:47 p.m.
Subject: Update

Keep the faith, Ann, and count the surgery as a weight loss :)

Colleen

Hug Everyone You Know

Since the consult, I had been trying not to be nervous. My stomach had not been fooled. I had been avoiding phone calls. Just saying the words, repeating the script, exhausted my attempts to remain optimistic and seemingly brave. I broadened my e-mail list to evade the telephone conversations. With only one message to write, I could plan my words carefully, fuss with semantics and syntax, and reply to any responses with a few lines of witty humor. This way, I did not have to hear the words spoken out loud and get so scared.

I could not, however, elude my girls, Mom, my sisters, or my dear, chatty friend and former college roommate, Renee, who now lived in Chicago. To them I was forced to relay the consult conversation with Dr. Axelrod and go over my surgery plan, recovery expectations, and treatment options. I spoke to Mary for a connection with oncologists at nearby Memorial Sloan Kettering's Commack facility or Stony Brook University Hospital.

There were so many unknowns. My right breast should heal and be "cosmetically appealing," according to Dr. Axelrod—but I wondered if a dimpled scar was considered cosmetically appealing.

Mom showed me her scars. The scar line was long, starting at the upper side of the breast and traveling across and downward toward her armpit. The deep dent where they'd taken out the tumor looked like a tight stitch in the middle of the blended incision. Under her arm, where twenty nodes were removed, was another long line scar. It sat as a reminder that she had to be careful of any hand or arm scratches or trauma. Without those lymph nodes, the tiniest infection could jeopardize her health.

"Your scars won't be as deep or long," Mom said, seeing that I was about to cry. "The new sentinel node and improved surgical procedures will leave much smaller scars."

Mom added that radiation therapy was the easiest part of her treatment. It took more time to drive to the facility and undress than to lay on the table and get zapped for a few seconds. It had given her a few skin burns and she'd felt tired toward the end of the six-week session, but it was a lot easier than chemotherapy.

The chemo options haunted me. On one hand, I thought that while I was in this cancer battle mode, I should just do it and be all that more certain it would never come back—kill anything suspicious and end up with a clean slate. But the thought of being purposely poisoned scared me. I worried for my girls and my husband. How would I be able to keep up with home and work? I was sick with the thought of not being in control of my own body.

Vanity was a vice no one could have accused me of before now. Over the years, I had morphed my hippie stylings into a tidy appearance. I continued to color my wild crop of curls to mimic youth and kept the unibrow and lip hairs under control. But I never had learned to use a hair dryer, nor did I spend time shaping and polishing my nails. Lipstick and an occasional swipe of the mascara brush were it for my makeup arsenal.

I blamed the weak beauty skills on my dad. As teenagers, my sisters and I had to dodge our father when we experimented with eye shadows and blush. If caught before we managed to get out the door, he would hold our face in one big hand and wipe the colors off our eyes with a damp thumb, saying, "My girls are too beautiful for all this paint."

Since the biopsy, though, I'd been looking more closely at my fallen face and lined neck. I never thought of myself as beautiful, just good-looking enough. I had been tall and sturdy through my adult years. Throughout my forties, however, I had steadily gained weight despite numerous diet plans and weight loss schemes. Now I looked older and sallower than I had one month earlier. The only surviving body parts that seemed to be ageless were my breasts. Now they were going to be ruined.

Vanity was creeping in.

chapter seven

Distractions

From: Mommy
To: Hallie
Date: Friday, February 16, 2007 at 8:12 p.m.
Subject: Kingston Weekend

We will meet you in Kingston tomorrow morning about 9/9:30-ish. We got a cheap hotel room for the night. Looking forward to some fun. Love you.

Mommy

~

From: Hallie
To: Mommy
Date: Friday, February 16, 2007 at 9:40 p.m.
Subject: Kingston Weekend

Yay! Can't wait to see you.

Hallie

Hug Everyone You Know

We drove to Kingston, a little town just north of New York City, not too far from New Paltz. Hallie's roller derby team was skating in an outdoor roller derby exhibition. The team had made a float for the town parade promoting some special event.

It didn't make much sense to hold a parade and outdoor women's roller derby bout in the middle of freezing February. But I needed a distraction and was willing to go anywhere. Kingston was anywhere. Besides, it was a great excuse to see Hallie.

Women's roller derby was enjoying a revival. Several loosely organized teams had sprouted up in a number of American cities and sleepy towns in recent years. Although it did not appear to be as rough as it had been some forty years ago, nor as sexy as it was when Raquel Welch portrayed it in *Kansas City Bomber,* it was extremely fast and the girls looked fierce. They also sported fun derby names like "Octopussy Pounder" and "Sally Slammer" on their jerseys.

I would never have imagined that my sweet Hallie, who'd never had the heart for contact sport competition, would embrace roller derby, but she'd been invited to try out for the Hudson Valley Horrors after interviewing the team for an article. She had quickly learned to skate fast, block, and jam. Her derby name was Candy Catastrophe.

"It's a great workout, Mommy," she claimed. "And I feel terrific after a practice and bout."

"Don't break your neck!" I heard myself say. As time went by I was sounding more like my mother, who was always warning against worst-case scenarios. No one could simply suffer a bump or a bruise; it always had to be a dire outcome, like a broken neck or death.

The women skated loudly. Hallie remained upright despite my vision of compound fractures. I had to admit, she did skate well, especially considering she was a novice and it was freezing cold on the asphalt parking lot. They were just a fun group of women having a great afternoon, nothing catastrophic about it.

Matt and I had a wonderful weekend with our girl, far away from cancer and surgery.

Back at home, everything felt stagnant. The house remained too tidy and clean. Throw blankets were folded and neatly draped on the back of the couch. The floor was swept clean of crumbs and cat dander. I was avoiding multistep dinner preps, which robbed the kitchen of its usual inviting aromas. The TV and stereo were kept to near mute levels.

I muddled through my workdays. My take-home files remained cold in the car overnight; I didn't have the attention span to tackle the tedium in the evening. Nothing was getting done! I did not want to talk about, read, or think about surgery, cancer, breasts, death, or taxes. (Matt was avoiding the elephant in the room by mumbling about preparing the taxes early.) Bringing the subject to the forefront made it too real, yet the continued silence exhausted me. Sleep could not find me.

I found a buried bag of yarn while clearing out Sara's

closet. She was living her independent life in Brooklyn, but boxes of CDs, forgotten shoes, and rolls of posters still lay in a chaotic pile in her closet.

Slender knitting needles stuck out from the yarn bag. They held together an unfinished gray mitten. I found my crochet needle stabbed in a ball of chocolate-brown yarn. Perhaps doing something with my hands would keep me distracted in this silent tomb.

Sara had taught herself to knit after giving up on my limited instruction of double and single crochet stitches. She'd concluded that crocheting was too simple since I didn't know how to make anything more than a four-sided shape.

My great-grandmother had taught me to crochet in hopes that I would continue the family pattern for doilies and tablecloths. My mother had been a dutiful child and learned to crochet and knit by her grandmother's toil, but she hadn't found it necessary or pleasant to teach her daughters. Besides, doilies had fallen out of home decor fashion by that point. Mom had kept a hutch drawer full of ancient doilies to use as emergency church hats while frantically getting four little girls out the door for early morning mass.

When Great-Grandma visited, she took it upon herself to hand my sisters and me a thick crochet needle and make us practice chains and single crochet stitches on coarse rug yarn. She was a tough taskmaster and communicated with exasperated Sicilian commands. If we missed a stitch or pulled the yarn unevenly, she would grab the sad chains and yank everything out. She *tsk-tsked* her tongue in her toothless mouth and redid the stitches within inches of our noses.

Although I stuck with the instructions longer than my

sisters did, I was never skilled or worthy enough to crochet beyond a pile of 3x5-inch granny squares. Maybe it was time to rededicate myself to the craft.

I stopped at the fabric store and browsed the aisles of yarns and do-it-yourself crocheting pamphlets. After some deliberation, I decided to crochet a scarf—a long, not-too-wide scarf in a happy shade that could be slip-knotted around my neck. Crocheting a scarf would be a practical project I could use to keep my head and hands busy and squelch the silence.

Coincidently, pink, breast cancer's mascot color, was truly my favorite color. My mother had assigned each of her four daughters a color of dress at birth. From that day forward we marched into church and relatives' homes for the holiday celebrations in similar jackets, dresses, and ankle socks in our assigned color. Pink was mine. I never grew out of it.

I chose a skein in a muted pink shade with frays of twisted yarn that gave the thin string added dimension. That night, after cleaning the kitchen post-dinner, I sat on the couch with a small canvas bag containing the new ball of yarn and my crochet needle. Petie nuzzled next to me, and we simultaneously breathed a contented sigh.

Finger memory immediately snapped into play. It flowed without my having to think, plan, or fuss over it. Crocheting, as I'd hoped it would, quieted my rambling thoughts and gave me a respite from the day's work. This was much better than sitting at the computer searching through cancer treatments and the multitude of possible situations.

Matt and I had to leave the house for most of Saturday; the realtor had scheduled another open house. We left Petie with Matt's mother. She enjoyed the little dog, who was content to curl up next to her on the couch.

Late in the afternoon, the realtor called to report that only two customers had come to tour the house. Frustrating.

Instead of going home, we met up with our friends Pam and Nick in Sayville. Pam reported that she had to be proactive with her bone health due to a recent osteoporosis diagnosis. Worse yet, our fun-loving friend Colleen now had to have a bone biopsy.

"It doesn't look good," Pam said. "This may be terminal."

"You can't say that until you absolutely know," Nick replied.

I couldn't find words.

To add to the dismal day, we saw *Letters from Iwo Jima* at the movie theater. It was a powerful saga that confirmed that no matter whose side you are on, war sucks. No one plans a life taken out of their control by the circumstances surrounding them. A terminal prognosis destroys the quiet fabric of everyday life, but war destroys the innocent in its path.

I was dealing with what should be a disruption, not a disaster. I should be grateful.

chapter eight

The Last Supper

From: Mom
To: Sara
Date: Saturday, February 24, 2007 at 1:10 a.m.
Subject: Dinner on Sunday

We will be in the city Sunday night, the 25th. Daddy's boss gave us the company credit card for dinner. Come!

~

From: Sara
To: Mom
Date: Saturday, February 24, 2007 at 1:25 a.m.
Subject: Dinner on Sunday

Ooooooo! Are we going someplace fancy and delicious?

I set up my aloof cat, Willow, with a clean litter box and enough food and water for two days. Petie stayed with

Matt's mom. Matt and I took an afternoon train into the city and checked into a hotel close by NYU Hospital.

Matt's CEO, JR, gave him the company credit card so we could go out for a nice dinner—the Last Supper. He recommended the Blue Water Grill in Union Square. Sara planned to meet us at six o'clock.

JR was especially sympathetic. His wife had suffered through brain cancer and succumbed three years ago. His grown children were attentive and consoling through her illness and death. He remained connected to his work, family, and home, but at the end of the day, the widowed man seemed lost and lonely.

If I should perish from this plight, I worried for my girls, my parents, and a long list of relations and friends, but I feared most for Matt. He would not be good as a lone rogue. He would need a good woman to keep him from being swallowed up by squalor or drinking himself beyond depression. He would need someone who would keep his passions fired. If I was beyond saving, I would need enough time to search for someone who would find him as endearing as I did, even though I would be very pissed off to have to do it.

Dinner at the Blue Water Grill was spectacular. Sara joined us for a sampling of oysters from different regions, each with its own distinctive taste. As expected, we decided our local Blue Point oysters were the plumpest and sweetest. Striped bass, seared scallops, and blackened tuna were complemented by two bottles of wine. We enjoyed the evening laughing at retold stories and eavesdropping on a neighbor's simmering table. Matt and Sara sampled shots of single malt scotch while I stirred a splash of Sambuca into my espresso.

Espresso! What was I thinking? I had to get up early in the morning. I stayed up most of the night with a muted late movie flickering in the darkened hotel room. I crocheted another scarf.

chapter nine

Surgical Circus

Monday, February 26, 2007

At seven thirty in the morning we took a cab to St. Vincent's Hospital on 12th Street to get my sentinel nodes dyed and radiated. St. Vincent's was one of the oldest hospitals on Manhattan Island, complete with familiar Catholic school beige brick walls and saints looking after all who stepped through the doors.

We took the elevator to the third floor to meet the young radiologist whom Dr. Axelrod held in such high esteem. Matt was directed to sit in the waiting room and sip the first brew of coffee. I changed into an examination gown. The doctor met me in his office. While perusing my file, he robotically explained the purpose and procedure.

". . . and the injection is inserted into the areola . . ."

I sat up. "What?"

He looked up from his thick, horned-rimmed glasses. "Please pull down the right side of your gown, slightly." He leaned over his desk and marked the right side of my chest with a sharpie. "Yes," he continued, scribbling in the file, "the areola, nipple. It is painful. Most patients report a nine or ten on a scale of one to ten." He looked up at me for the first time. "Don't move, since I like to get this done in one shot. You will have to lie still for fifteen minutes as the dye moves to the nodes."

I numbly followed him to the procedure room, where I was directed to lie on my back on a hard surgical table next to the gamma radiation camera. A large nurse smiled kindly at me while positioning my right arm above my head—finally, compassionate eye contact in this stark place.

"Try not to move, dear."

The doctor leaned over my right breast. I could smell the sour milk from his morning coffee. He plunged the needle into the edge of the nipple. He was right: It hurt! Really, really hurt! I passed out, only able to hear a distant voice commanding me, "Breathe! Open your eyes!"

A whiff of ammonia brought me back long enough to mutter, "I'll be back later."

I opened my eyes to Matt holding my hand and explaining to the nurse that the fainting happened all the time and was nothing to worry about. Thankfully, the procedure was successful the first time. I got up, dressed, and was whisked to the NYU Cancer Center on 34th Street for the wire placement.

"Don't tell me what, why, or how you do this," I told the doctor, "Just get it done and ignore me."

The doctor was amused by this request but soon called in for assistance once my color drained and I became unresponsive. While a sonogram beamed the position of the tumor, the wire was thrust into my breast. It would eventually guide the surgeon to the tumor's exact location.

Once lucid, they had me stand up for a mammogram to prove the wire was properly placed.

"Perfect pictures!" the doctor announced. With the wire taped to my chest (perhaps over the sharpie marking) and films in hand, I was taken to ambulatory surgery at the hospital. The clock read ten forty-five when I entered the lobby. My surgery was scheduled for noon.

The waiting room was filled with restless patients and their loved ones. I was afraid to move my arm, fearing I might dislodge the now throbbing wire. After I'd been waiting two hours, Dr. Axelrod found me and reported that an emergency had backed up the operating room schedule. A familiar migraine crept in within an hour. The fluorescent lights blinded me, and I abandoned any hope of reading or crocheting. The thick air of the anxiety-filled room triggered a nauseating aura. The throbbing wound where the wire entered my skin only exacerbated the pounding discomfort. I reasoned with myself that this day would be the worst and it was already almost over.

I remained quiet, knowing that no amount of complaining was going to make anything move any faster. Matt had had enough by three o'clock. I had grown paler, and the migraine was hammering me relentlessly. He reported to a nurse at the window that I might be running a fever now that I was sufficiently dehydrated.

Suddenly, everything moved forward. I was sent to a darkened room where a long vein hunt in my arm ensued.

Finally, dripped fluids coursed through my body, alleviating the headache and the throb in my chest. Questions were answered, forms signed, and I received a reassuring pat from every attending nurse, the anesthetist, and a nun. Finally, at five-thirty, I was shuttled into the OR, placed in a crucifix position, and directed to count backward from one hundred. I meant to ask why one hundred. Was it going to take that long to fall asleep? But I didn't get to ask because I was out before managing to say anything.

I woke up retching. "All is well," reported a blurry nurse. "You did beautifully."

I didn't feel too beautiful, with a puddle of vomit in my lap and the world swirling around me.

Matt almost skipped in, all smiles. "Dr. Axelrod said she got it all—the tumor and the margins—and the nodes were clear!" He kissed me, relieved and exhilarated. "I called the girls and your mom. I told them you were fine."

It took extra time for my vitals to remain steady. I was the last patient out of the recovery room. Finally, upright and coherent, I was wheeled to the front lobby to meet a cab back to the hotel.

We took our time getting up in the morning and leaving for the train ride home. The winter air was crisp and clear. The traffic seemed to rumble, "Good morning!" I had to smile. What a beautiful day. I took it as a positive omen.

chapter ten

Homecoming

Finally home. Home, where I could change into flannel pajamas, draw the curtains, and bury myself under thick blankets for a long deserved sleep. The pain was bothersome, but the Vicodin had made me nauseous. I just needed to lie down. I planned to call the girls and Mom later in the evening.

But something was wrong as soon as I stepped into the house. The pyramid of houseplants that sat in the front window was toppled. Their leaves, roots, and soil were scattered through the living room and into the dining room. The cat's dry food crunched under my boots as I made my way into the kitchen. The napkin holder and salt and pepper shakers were on the floor. Newspaper pages lay disheveled on the coffee table in the family room. Even the folded throw blankets looked jumbled on the back of the couch.

I never had trouble leaving our cat, Willow, alone for two days. She had never damaged anything! She sauntered up from the basement grousing, ignoring my plea for an explanation. Our dog, Petie, entered the house on high alert. He quickly surveyed the downstairs rooms and frantically trotted upstairs, only to quickly scamper back down. He looked at Willow, who turned her tail at him, and then looked at Matt and me. Something had happened, and Petie needed to know what. I, however, did not need to know—not at the moment. What I needed was my bed.

I left Matt to investigate and clean up. Petie followed me upstairs to my bedroom, only to rush back down. He did this several times, torn between lying next to me for a cozy nap or finding out what had happened.

After fifteen minutes of this, Matt walked into the bedroom with Petie. "Keep him with you. There's a squirrel in the house."

Squirrel was one of the ten words Petie recognized. Although he was supposed to be a smart Jack Russell Terrier, he had proven to be a dim-witted soul. He could not problem solve as readily as expected, nor did he learn from prior experiences. His backyard nemeses were the squirrels that stole the birdseed, dug millions of shallow holes, and enjoyed tormenting him. When Petie spied them from the back door, he would yip and jump straight up and down at the window until the door was slid open, at which point he would burst out of the door on a mad chase. The varmints would sprint to the closest tree, leaving Petie grounded with his high-pitched bark. Some of them had the audacity to chatter back to him and throw acorns at his head. They had incredible aim.

Petie whimpered and pawed at the closed bedroom door. I called for him to join me in the bed, but he could not stay still knowing his sworn enemy was in his home. Finally, Matt came upstairs to report.

"I don't know how it got in, but it could not find its way back out. Apparently, this squirrel spent the weekend with the cat. There is squirrel shit everywhere. Willow is happily napping on the couch, looking no worse for the wear."

Matt found the traumatized squirrel huddled in the front closet. He swept it out the front door, allowing it to limp its way into the bushes. The next morning, Petie bolted out the back door and quickly caught the dazed squirrel as it was venturing to the bird feeder. With a mighty shake, he killed the creature, dropped it, and proudly came inside for a well-earned breakfast.

Yikes! I did not want to take this drama as an omen of what was yet to come.

From: Antoinette
To: My Everyone
Date: Tuesday, February 27, 2007 at 8:22 p.m.
Subject: I'm fine

The worst is over. It was a very long day, but it is done. The initial results are very positive. The nodes were negative for any cancer. I'll have a full pathology report next Tuesday. It looks good. I think that whatever treatment needs to be done will be minimal.

I appreciate your thoughts, prayers, and positive energies sent my way. Believe me, it truly helps to know that I have so many rooting for me. I'm truly blessed.

So, now to move forward. I am going back to work on Thursday, the house is still up for sale, and it smells like spring. Be well.

Hug everyone you know.
Ann

~

From: Renee
To: Antoinette
Date: Tuesday, February 27, 2007 at 8:48 p.m.
Subject: I'm fine

Oh, I am so glad it is over; you sound positive, just as my old roomie always does. I just know you are going to sail through the rest of this and really be sailing in a few short months. We are still coming to New York in the spring, so we will see you soon.

Renee

~

From: Dan and Coll
To: Antoinette
Date: Tuesday, February 27, 2007 at 8:49 p.m.
Subject: I'm fine

We're relieved and more than happy. We will have lots to celebrate on I-Night.

chapter eleven

The Interview

From: Antoinette
To: Colleen
Date: Friday, March 2, 2007 at 9:02 p.m.
Subject: Just Checking

Hi honey,
Just checking to hear how you are holding up. Mary told me she assumed your identity and got your insurance and appointments squared away. Amazing how she can sound so authoritative and get so much done. It's a gift. Know that you can have wine and beer while waiting for things to happen. Also, know that you are in excellent hands at Sloan Kettering. More importantly you are loved, and the power of prayer and positive energies will make a huge difference.

I had a good day. I interviewed at Remsenburg-Speonk today. I stuffed my boobs into a sports bra. Some protesting ensued in getting them in and looking even. No one was the wiser. (At least no one mentioned it, although, now thatI think about it, no one would mention it. They are all polite.) No matter, I got the job! By September all this drama will be done, these babies should be perky, and I will be doing work I am really good at and proud to do.

Happy birthday to your beautiful Devon. Hope all of you got to eat cake!

Hug everyone you know.
Ann

The interview at the Remsenburg-Speonk School was first thing Friday morning. I tucked my very sore breast into a wireless sports bra that provided very little anti-gravity support. I pulled on panty hose, zipped up a power skirt, and shrugged on the coordinating suit jacket. With a bit of makeup to hide the dark eye circles, sticky mousse worked into my hair, and lipstick, I appeared my sturdy, practical self.

I felt a wave of relief walking into the familiar school building, carrying my portfolio. I knew this elementary school. My girls attended here. I volunteered on the PTA board. Matt coached the softball team for a few seasons.

Fourteen years prior, Matt and I had found ourselves bursting out of our little cottage in Sayville. At the time, I worked with many families on the east end of Long Island and had learned that not all of the quaint east-end hamlets were summer party scenes. There were many year-round residents that quietly boasted low taxes, excellent schools, great beaches, and fishing. All this was just twenty-five miles east of our Sayville home base. We were able to afford more house there (a handyman special, but I had Matt as my resident handyman), and the local elementary school featured one class per grade and an abundance of resources. The small classes, caring staff, and friendly atmosphere were key for each of my daughters, but essential for Robyn.

Robyn's early language development was always a half step behind. I was incredibly fortunate to work in a therapeutic preschool that offered staff day care and provided Robyn the extra attention and structure she needed. Being a speech therapist that specialized in early childhood development also helped. However, being Mom and speech therapist were difficult dual roles. One cannot effectively therapize their own. Robyn's scores never qualified her for services, but I saw the splinter skills she was using to compensate.

When I registered Robyn for kindergarten in Remsenburg, I was able to talk to the director of special education, Jan Achilich. Within the first few months of school, Robyn joined the speech improvement group to hone her phonemic and early academic skills.

By the third grade, Robyn's auditory processing "quirks" were making focusing, as well as reading fluency and comprehension, extremely difficult. Being a no-nonsense kid, she worked very hard during the school day. She brought home all of her textbooks and notebooks to ensure she had everything she needed to finish incomplete classwork and the regular homework. Every afternoon she came home from school short-tempered and in need of a forty-five-minute nap.

Robyn was far from failing, but she needed help. She was tested and classified as a student with a learning disability. This afforded her additional resources and modifications.

Learning became so much more accessible. The intimate care and attention she received in those early elementary school years enabled her to gain the foundations of reading and writing, and become a successful student. While attending this little elementary school, she developed learning strategies that would follow her through her academic career—and the rest of her life. Robyn graduated high school on the honor roll and eventually graduated from college with honors. I had always been proud of my tough baby girl, and credited Jan Achilich and the Remsenburg-Speonk Elementary School teachers with saving her education, self-esteem, and future.

Through the years, I had maintained a very amenable professional relationship with Jan. It was by sheer coincidence that we both attended a transitional early-intervention meeting in Remsenburg, and Jan mentioned that my children's former elementary school was in search of a dual-certified special education/speech therapist experienced with very disabled children. They were looking to hire for the next school year. I nominated myself.

The frigid morning made spring seem so far away. I said hello to the teachers I recognized and caught up with the friendly school secretary, Debbie Martel. Before I headed into the superintendent's office, Debbie confirmed arrangements for my children's author/illustrator group's school visit, which was scheduled in a few weeks. The event was the culmination of a school and home-reading initiative. Local children's authors and illustrators would set up tables cluttered with their books and accessories in the gymnasium, and children, parents, and teachers would get to chat with them, purchase their books, and have them personally signed. The occasion also gave the artists a means to showcase their work. They were terrific events.

The interview with Jan and the principal, Kathy Salomone, quickly morphed into a comfortable conversation. Within twenty minutes, Jan announced that I was hired. The business office had a salary and benefits packet to be reviewed at my leisure. I could finish the written application and paperwork any time, since the budget vote and board approval would not be scheduled for a few months.

I did not need to mention cancer. It would be a memory by the time September rolled around. I left the little school with a big name for my soon-to-be previous job with the biggest grin. I had not been able to smile that broadly since January. Everything was falling into place. My health was getting under control, and now I'd been handed a new job with work I was proud to do. It suddenly smelled like spring. This cancer was certain to be a short detour.

From: Colleen
To: Antoinette
Date: Saturday, March 3, 2007 at 7:50 a.m.
Subject: Just Checking

You make me chuckle, my friend. I picked up some sport bras from Kmart myself. (I might be sick, but I am still cheap.) You got the job! Now that is a good day. So glad to hear you could get the "girls" under control. I am feeling that my day was good as well since at least getting appointments moves me forward in getting something done about this mess. I will keep you posted.

XXXOOO Colleen

Colleen's plight was not that easy. She had passed all of the stages and gone straight to Stage IV breast cancer. What she thought were normal aches and pains, perhaps carpal tunnel, turned out to be masses eating her bones and threatening her lymph system. Mary wrestled with Colleen's insurance carrier and arranged for her to see an excellent doctor at Memorial Sloan Kettering Cancer Center. There was a nearby campus in Commack, so whatever had to get done could get done close to home.

How had this happened to a young woman (forty-four) who had always been vigilant with exams and mammograms? Her daughter was just turning sixteen, and her little boy was still little—ten years old. Colleen's mother had succumbed to cancer too young. This was not supposed to happen!

I told myself I should be grateful. I faced an excellent prognosis. I should be glad that this was happening now, with me strong and healthy and my kids not living at home. They would not have to see me go through whatever I had to get through. I had experienced no symptoms, and there was no pain to endure. I believed it would all work out, with merely short-term disruptions along the way. The mammography screening had done its job: identified a tumor early, before any damage was incurred. I had no business feeling sorry for myself. I should not be so anxious, especially since my friend was, as she put it, "wrestling alligators."

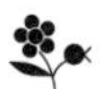

My follow-up appointment with my surgeon was coming up. I resolved that I did not want to put myself at risk for this again. I should not argue against an aggressive route—save a mastectomy—while in this fight mode. Perhaps my ovaries should be removed to reduce the raging estrogen that fed the cancer, and I should undergo radiation to zap any microscopic leftover cells—even chemotherapy to make sure any stray cancer cells would not survive. I should not take the easiest way out just to save myself the discomfort. And I had to get serious about losing weight. Giving cancer an opportunity to crop up again was not an option.

From: Antoinette
To: My Everyone
Date: Tuesday, March 6, 2007 at 6:45 p.m.
Subject: Report card

We are back from the surgeon. I got an A- on my pathology report! Small, clear margins, clear nodes, and officially Stage 1 type of tumor. And, as a bonus, the genetic testing came back negative. For the over-achiever, the minus is there because the damn thing is still cancer. It's OK. I'll take it. My surgeon expects that radiation therapy (4–6 weeks) and hormone management (hoping it won't damage my sweet disposition) will be prescribed. I have an appointment with the same oncologist my mom sees at the nearby Memorial Sloan Kettering Cancer Center in Commack. How lucky is that, to have a state of the art facility so close by! I want to get this over with ASAP. Summer is coming. I had been told that I will be tattooed for the radiation therapy. My girls called with several suggestions.

Thank you all for your positive energies and prayers. I am so encouraged by all of the sincerity and love.

Hug everyone you know.
Antoinette

~

From: Dan & Coll
To: Antoinette
Date: Tuesday, March 6, 2007 at 8:55 p.m.
Subject: Report card

That is wonderful news!! Let's celebrate this weekend.

Coll & Dan

~

The appointment with Dr. Axelrod went well. My breast and arm were healing and, so far, I had experienced no lymphedema symptoms (excess fluids buildup due to the lymph nodes removal). The preliminary pathology report stated that the tumor was .98 centimeters, estrogen receptive, and the margins and nodes were negative for cancer. A final report was forthcoming. Dr. Axelrod was confident it was no more than a Stage 1 cancer. Since the tumor was under a centimeter and there was no node or margin involvement, a short course of radiation therapy would most likely be prescribed. I would also have to take Tamoxifen to suppress estrogen. Like it or not, menopause would be forced upon my body and overall good nature.

As instructed, I made an appointment with an oncologist. I decided to go with Dr. Sheren at Memorial Sloan Kettering Cancer Center in Commack. Why travel into the city when I had an excellent facility on Long Island? Mom had seen Dr. Sheren for her follow-up visits and had been very happy with the smart, friendly doctor.

Mary helped me make sure my insurance covered the expenses. All reports would be sent to MSKCC in plenty of time for my March 28th appointment. Three more weeks of waiting.

chapter twelve

I-Night

Dan and Coll were hosting our monthly International Dinner Party Night (I-Night). In 1986, Matt's high school clamming buddies found themselves back in our hometown territory after some ten years of college, defining careers in various parts of the country, marriage, and home buying. I had been part of the post–high school crowd since Matt and I had gotten together at age seventeen, but it was the men who shared a tight bond. In our early married years, we found it difficult and expensive to go out to our usual haunts together, so we decided to set a monthly Saturday night aside to cook and share an amazing meal. We round-robined our meal course roles. The hosts chose a theme, region, or country and took on the main course. Another couple prepared appetizers and brought regional beer. The soup cooks brought wine and the fourth couple handled a dessert and appropriate after-dinner cordials. Our original agreement included tackling recipes we had never tried before.

As the years sped forward, our families expanded, homes were bought and sold, jobs were left and found. We saw each other through child-rearing issues and joys, and the loss of parents. I-Nights continued, although there was a month or two that lapsed due to any number of scheduling conflicts. On those nights, through the evening and into the early morning hours, we solved the world's problems, shared our kids' latest antics, and discussed the challenges and merits of the chosen recipes. We cooked and ate around the world, honored favored chefs, and collected cookbooks and clever gadgets. It was always fun, always satisfying for soul and stomach, and always worth the effort.

This month, Dan and Coll had chosen New Orleans Mardi Gras cuisine. We were a month late with this celebration, but the region was so delicious and fun. Celebrating was in order. I had to come up with a dessert, the hardest course. I was a skilled cook but no pastry chef. Desserts require careful measuring, true attention to step sequence, and a watchful eye. There is also an artistic hand required in order for desserts to look pretty and appetizing. I had a tiny plastic baby from someone's baby shower buried in the junk drawer. I decided to bake it into a King Cake and declare the finder the lucky king or queen of the party.

It took me all afternoon to bake the cake into a ring. It did not look even. The glaze dripped too quickly off the spoon. I decided to put the finishing glaze and colored sugar on just before serving it. Coll, the master baker of the group, could help me get the glaze to cooperate. I spent the rest of the afternoon cleaning sticky counters and floor.

Matt and I arrived promptly at six. Dan made room in the refrigerator to fit the lopsided cake. Before settling into our I-Night routine, my wine glass was filled and I gave a brief synopsis of the surgery and the probable treatment protocol.

"It's all going to work out fine," Matt repeated.

Fluke, who shared my aversion to vein punctures and gory details, put down his beer to give me a tight, loving hug. We were done talking about cancer. We had a tremendous meal to devour. Coll got the glaze to drip just right on my King Cake, and, in keeping with true I-Night tradition, taste triumphed over presentation.

It was Matt, in the end, who pulled the plastic baby out of his mouth. Lucky man.

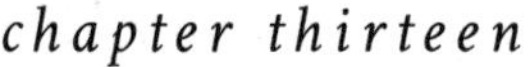

chapter thirteen

Added Agita

Robyn's spring break landed on the worst travel weekend. Snow buried upstate New York, fouling the roads and forcing everyone to stay indoors. But Robyn decided to get into her not-so-bright friend's car and follow the storm south to Long Island. What the hell was she thinking? My nerves wrapped around my chest, making it difficult to breathe, let alone follow a conversation with a county coordinator who was complaining, once again, about a parent asking for too many services. I raced home to aggressively vacuum in hopes of distracting my worry.

Robyn finally called from outside of Albany saying that the New York State Thruway was closed. The storm was as bad as I had predicted.

"I guess it was a stupid idea to drive in this," she admitted.

I told her to use the emergency credit card to get a room in the nearest motel and stay put until the storm passed. When she got home, I planned to firmly explain that I was in no shape to deal with her adventures. She would have to lead a practical, safe life until I was recovered from all this cancer nonsense. She called back an hour later to report they'd found a Motel 6 close to a prison and been lucky to get a room because the storm had stranded so many travelers. I hollered loud and clear that she and her not-so-bright friend were to use all of the locks on the door and windows and *not* leave their room until they checked out.

"Don't even go outside to use the vending machine! I don't care how hungry you are!" I shouted.

It must have worked, because her not-so-bright friend's mother called later to relay that the girls were too scared to leave the room until the morning. I ached to bear hug Robyn—and then shake her with all my might.

Although I had tried to keep my situation low-key, word got around. A social worker had been calling regularly to check up on me. She was concerned, and, being a cancer survivor herself, she replayed her harrowing experiences. I politely listened, leaning the phone receiver against my ear and pumping my right arm over my head while checking my e-mail. I marveled at how she monologued her plight so fluently. She had been running a breast cancer support group and insisted the camaraderie would do me good. I finally agreed but was determined not to go alone.

From: Antoinette
To: Colleen
Date: Monday, March 19, 2007 at 8:45 p.m.
Subject: Support Group

So this was bound to happen. A very nice social worker I work with is a breast cancer survivor. She had a double mastectomy, chemo, and reconstruction surgery. She claims her new breasts are perkier at age sixty than when she was fifteen. I can't verify even though she offered to show me. She is very active in the breast cancer community and now heads up a support group. She has been relentless in inviting me to attend her meetings. I am reluctant since, well, I'm feeling relatively lucky for the type of cancer I have and don't think I really fit in with women who may really be sick. But she is a very kind person and insists everyone needs support. I don't want to pass her up again. This next meeting has a doctor coming in to talk about exercise and keeping healthy during and after treatment. I thought if I could go with my good friend, who happens to have cancer as well, we could both get something out of it, even if it's only a night out on a "school" night. It's free, and we are under no obligation to continue. It's April 7 in Nesconset; I'll drive.

I am still feeling this is unreal. Except for the scars, I kind of forget I am on this journey. Even my regular bras fit! My appointment at Sloan is next week, so reality is looming. Being forced into menopause is feeling scary as well. Maybe we can be menopausal together. I just hope I don't get too loony. It will really scare Matt. Talk soon. Enjoy the spring day.

Hug everyone you know.
Ann

~

From: Colleen
To: Antoinette
Date: Tuesday, March 20, 2007 at 11:48 a.m.
Subject: Support Group

Ah, just when I think the burden is getting too heavy for my shoulders, my ten-year-old cutie comes home from school with a big hug and my friend comes up with a fabulous idea. Sounds like a date. Send me the particulars.

I am thinking that overnight menopause is a "Get Out of Jail Free" card to be moody and gain weight. The whole depression thing does not work for me, though. There are far too many things to laugh about in this world. Besides, we are way too skippy cute to turn into ranting lunatics. And while your news is "good" in the grand scheme of cancer, any cancer just plain bites the big one! XXOO

It was official. Colleen's bone biopsy reported an aggressive Stage IV metastasized breast cancer. The pain in her neck, back, and hands was the result of the bones breaking down. Her oncologist proposed a plan of hormone therapy, pain management, and regular Zometa infusions to mitigate the bone deterioration—no surgery since treating the whole body was paramount. This seemed like such a drastic finding considering she felt "skippy good."

"You are a very beautiful, healthy, forty-four-year-old woman who just happens to have breast cancer that spread to your bones," the oncologist told her. "Other than that, you are fine."

Shit!

~

From: Antoinette
To: Mary
Date: Tuesday, March 20, 2007 at 1:48 p.m.
Subject: Colleen

Did you get Colleen's email? Does this plan sound as if they can only keep her comfortable as the cancer eats her? Is hormone therapy really that effective? Isn't there anything else? I'm confused and upset.

~

From: Mary
To: Antoinette
Date: Tuesday, March 20, 2007 at 2:19 p.m.
Subject: Colleen

Ann, Stage IV cancer is very serious. Statistics show that the five-year survival rate is less than 20 percent. Hormone therapy is just one tool in an arsenal of weapons. Eventually, chemotherapy will be needed, but so much depends on how she handles a therapy and how the cancer responds. Chemotherapy destroys cancer cells as well as healthy cells. Although chemo treatment has gotten better at targeting primary cancer cells, there is always collateral damage. The good news is that if you had to choose a breast metastasis, bone is the most manageable. Most specialists will tell you that managing this late stage cancer is the goal, not the cure. But it is going to be a fight. Colleen needs to be aggressive at this time for sure, but some women just can't handle aggressive therapy over a long period of time.

I wish the news was more hopeful. The next two years will be telling. For now, her friends and family need to be positive and supportive.

This is a completely different situation from you and from Mommy. When Mommy was diagnosed eight years ago, almost all women in your age group would get a round of chemotherapy even though a small percentage were actually at a risk for recurrence. Today there is a new test, the MammaPrint, that can predict if chemotherapy is really necessary. The radiation and hormone therapies may suffice. I am sure it was ordered, and the results will be used to guide your treatment. Timing is everything, Ann. Six months ago, this test was not available. Lucky you! Cure is the norm in your case. I just wish it were so for Colleen. Let me know how your appointment goes next week.

Mary

~

Although relieved by the relative good news from the surgeon, I was offered only a projected treatment plan. I wanted the projecting to stop. My rambling imagination kept replaying in my head. I feared that if I said anything out loud, it might become real. The anxiety tightened my chest, and the fatigue made it difficult to keep up with work and cleaning the house each time a realtor called. Sleep evaded me. What had happened to my attention span? I started to crochet a bedspread in a loud orange-and-green pattern. It soon got too heavy to tote in my bag. I thought maybe I needed a pill. I knew I needed a plan.

On March 23, 2007, I sat packed tight on a 7:04 a.m. train into Penn Station. The early spring day required only a jacket—such a refreshing contrast from the walks up 34th Street in frosty February. Despite the promise of spring, the city moved quickly and loudly, not a friendly face in sight. I hurried along the streets, weaving around slower pedestrians, keeping ahead of the flowing shuffle. Once again, my stride stopped short at the large doors with *CANCER* sprawled over the header. The reality of walking around with cancer was still unreal. Soon enough, though, I would not be walking around with it. This was my last walk to NYUCC. I came to pick up the pathology slides and films, then catch a train back to the island, drop off the package to Memorial Sloan Kettering at Commack, and get in a half day of work.

On the train ride home, I schemed as to how and when I could resign from the agency. I did not want to have to face my supervisor's drama. I didn't want any of my coworkers to feel her wrath as the cases were shuffled. A fellow early-intervention teacher I frequently contracted might want the job. She could easily slip in and do the work. It was just that the position was difficult to be in when you had been on the family side of the business. Being in this coordinator position compromised the values I had believed in throughout my career. It was even harder to listen quietly to people who had little to no field experience complain and insult the contracted therapists and teachers.

If I needed an ovary removal or hysterectomy, I thought I could perhaps schedule it after Hallie's graduation, before the summer. I could get local early intervention contract work for the summer wherever "local" was going to be, since our house still stood with a "For Sale" sign on its threshold. Between surgery and radiation therapy (which should not be too bad), I could gracefully resign, citing that I needed to reevaluate my priorities and set new goals. I would not mention that I really needed to work in a more positive environment where my expertise and energy would be appreciated.

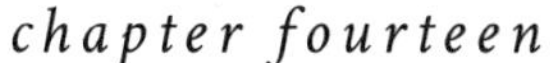

chapter fourteen

Damn It!

Dr. Sheren confidently shook my hand and offered Matt a warm smile. She said the tumor was invasive and there were calcifications. She explained that my age, the size of the tumor, and my family history put me at a greater risk for recurrence. She re-explained the report and the standards and answered our questions. I couldn't really understand her. She prescribed a CMF (cytoxan, methotrexate, fluorouracil) chemotherapy protocol—a mild cocktail that should do the trick. She talked about eight infusion sessions, one every three weeks, followed by a daily dose of radiation therapy. I asked more questions. Matt repeated the questions. It didn't matter. We did not hear anything.

The nurse came in with paperwork and tubes for a blood draw.

"Wait a minute," I said. "Maybe we should think about this. I was told that this cancer is not that involved."

Dr. Sheren was sorry the surgeon did not have the full report when I saw her last. She could order the MammaPrint but was not hopeful that it would result in a different scenario. She explained that Memorial Sloan Kettering had specific and successful procedures. Although we were welcome to explore other options, she strongly believed that the CMF and radiation therapies were the most effective and safest way to defeat this cancer.

She took my hand and smiled into my eyes. "Think about it. Call if you have any questions, but don't wait too long. You need to do something soon." She shook Matt's hand, smiled—the smile I would soon come to know—and repeated to him that we needed to decide soon.

We left armed with information brochures. Our heads swirled. We rode back to Remsenburg in anxious silence. I had the Authors and Illustrators Night at Remsenburg-Speonk that evening, so I had to get home, pack up my wares, and enthusiastically greet and sign books for my young fans. I did not want to think about chemotherapy, cancer, IVs, blood work, or nausea. The phone chirps were ignored.

At home, Matt sat at the kitchen table as I scurried about getting ready for the event. He browsed through the brochures and then finally broke down in sobs. "How are you going to do this?" he said between gulps. "You do so much, and you never react normally to any drugs."

He was right. In my very limited experience, my reactions to medicines were not listed on the two-page disclaimers. A half an antihistamine caused hallucinations worthy of an LSD trip. My first reaction to Demerol caused me to yank IVs and monitors off of my body, grab my strong husband by the neck, and demand that he to take me home despite the fact I was in active labor. There was also the constant problem of losing consciousness when a vein was punctured.

"Because I have to," was my only retort. This was my life. This cancer was supposed to be a bump in a long life road. I had promised myself that I would be as aggressive as necessary. So here it was—more aggressive than radiation, less drastic than a mastectomy: a middle-ground compromise. Matt would have to pick up the housekeeping slack, and I would have to manage work more efficiently. I knew his big problem was the idea of seeing me go through the infusions, the side effects, and, worst of all, the tears. He hated tears, especially mine.

I shouldered my bags and kissed him. "I can do this; you can do this. I don't want to go through this ever again. I'm calling the doctor in the morning."

Dr. Sheren's nurse had said I could come in at my convenience to talk. Impressive. Already, I loved this doctor's manner. She met me in a small examination room. Her lunch sat on the counter, uneaten. She explained (probably for the sixth time) that the CMF would be effective yet not as damaging as other chemotherapy treatments. I would have eight treatments in three-week intervals, to be followed by radiation therapy. I would not lose all my hair, and the nausea would be manageable. She would also add Ativan to my order to reduce my obvious anxiety. She ordered the MammaPrint but repeated that it probably would not sway the course of action. I signed papers, she checked her schedule, and we agreed to begin on April 10.

"You are a strong, healthy woman," she said with that

smile. "You will get through this and go on to live a long, healthy life."

I believed her.

From: Antoinette
To: My Everyone
Date: Wednesday, March 28, 2007 at 10:15 p.m.
Subject: An update

Well, the visit to the oncologist, Dr. Sheren, was . . . disappointing. Yes, Memorial Sloan Kettering is a beautiful and comfortable facility. You get the feeling they all know what they are doing. The final pathology report was not as glowing as the initial. The tumor is invasive, which puts me at a higher risk. It's still very curable. Dr. Sheren recommended radiation and hormone therapy, and a modified course of chemo. It's a lighter cocktail, and for those of you who know my ability to manage cocktails, a modified cocktail is about all I could tolerate. No hair loss, well at least no more than a thinning, and since my hair is so thick anyway, a little thinning won't be such a bad thing. I will keep my eyelashes and eyebrows (plucking and waxing regimes will have to continue) and no real physical side effects except for the fatigue thing. This is very curable and although a bigger bump than what I was banking on, it is just that, a bump. I am more interested in making sure this does not happen again. Recurrence is scarier than the initial journey. Getting this over and done with is the mission. Keeping healthy and my usual good-natured self, at least until my 103rd birthday, is the goal.

Again, everyone, thank you, thank you. Your prayers, positive energies, and well-wishing are truly a blessing.

Hug everyone you know.
Antoinette

~

From: Renee
To: Antoinette
Date: Wednesday, March 28, 2007 at 11:15 p.m.
Subject: An update

So you have a little more work to do than anticipated, but you'll do it well and kick the crap out of that thing. You'll be diligent and thorough and ask questions and get answers and do all the right things. I have complete faith. I will be visiting my family for Passover. Can I come see you? Gotta give you a huge hug!

Renee

I worried about my daughters. I spoke to each of them when I got back from the Authors and Illustrators Night. Matt had called them earlier, so there were no gasps or tears over the phone. We were all calm, and we resigned to fight the fight and then walk away. They were not accustomed to me being sick or physically compromised in any way. As for most supermoms, colds and headaches had to respond to an aspirin and/or inattention. The household would not function if I had a sick day, and it was always too much work to catch up from one, anyway. Up until now, I had never needed to take a sick day from my family.

I could hear the anxiety in each of their voices. They were not buying my overconfidence. Hallie said that maybe she shouldn't take an internship in New York City, and instead she should stay home to help. Robyn wondered if she should just come home. Sara felt helpless in not being able to be with me.

"No!" I told them all. I was not going to allow them to rearrange their lives. They were sweet and considerate and I love them more than life, but I would not allow them to sacrifice for this goddamn cancer! Still, I had to come up with something they could do so they wouldn't feel so lost.

~

From: Mom
To: Sara, Hallie, & Robyn
Date: Thursday, March 29, 2007 at 12:43 a.m.
Subject: An update

I am so glad I got to talk to each of you tonight. The chemo recommendation really threw me off. I honestly thought a few weeks of radiation and I'd be off the hook. Daddy is upset. He knows what a wimp I am when it comes to needles getting close to my arms. And then there is the proven fact that I do not respond to medications as expected. He is afraid I will grow weak and sick for seven or eight months. He may have to figure out the vacuum. I wouldn't mind surrendering the vacuum but would really be upset with the puking. I managed three pregnancies without one hurl. The doctor has a rainbow of drugs to help ease the anxiety during the infusion, BUT I may need something to help me deflect the puking. I am not sure if I can discuss cannabis with the doctor I just met. Would you girls be able to safely access a small stash for me or, better yet, know where to get some? Dad resurrected the ancient bong from our college days. It looks awful. I think he may have to venture into a "head" shop. Suggestions? I will send money for it. And don't tell Grandma. Don't tell your cousins either because Grandma will eventually find out through my sisters.

Love you more than you can know.
Mommy

~

From: Robyn
To: Mom
Date: Thursday, March 29, 2007 at 12:54 a.m.
Subject: An update

No problem, Mom. I can mail it in a cigar box. I'll add a couple of roach clips too, in case Dad can't get a bong.

Robyn

~

From: Sara
To: Mom
Date: Thursday, March 29, 2007 at 12:57 a.m.
Subject: An update

I'm on it! Don't get a bong that is small or cute. I'll call Dad at his office later today. I want to be sure you get the right stuff. Good night. Love you.

Sara

From: Hallie
To: Mommy
Date: Thursday, March 29, 2007 at 1:02 a.m.
Subject: An update

Cool! I have a friend who has a friend in Kingston. My other friend can give my friend a ride on Thursday. I can be home for the weekend. We can try it out together. Love you, Mommy.

From: Robyn
To: Mom
Date: Thursday, March 29, 2007 at 3:00 a.m.
Subject: An update

Hey Mom,
I have a better idea. Since you don't like to smoke, I could bake brownies. I have a very good recipe. I will mail them wrapped in the cigar box with the roach clips, too. Feel good!

Robyn

I had to admit, I did not expect such seamless resources and enthusiasm.

chapter fifteen

Therapy

I picked up Colleen on my way to the support group. We schemed that if we got uncomfortable, we could slip out at the break and head for the hotel bar. I had never been comfortable in group therapy with people I did not know. I did not like being asked to contribute or respond to a stranger's pain, or being told it was okay not to contribute or respond when it obviously wasn't. I was also uncomfortable with overzealous acknowledgments of accomplishments like not gaining three pounds in a week. Maybe this was why I found the Weight Watchers meetings so distasteful.

I had had positive experiences with grief support groups during the '80s and early '90s, however. My early intervention caseload was filled with babies and families who had the HIV/AIDS virus and/or the product of crack/cocaine addiction. The heartbreak and pain that existed in so many homes sapped all hope and energies. I had to attend too many funerals with closed tiny white coffins surrounded by perfumed lilies. At that time, I was fortunate to work for an agency that valued their teachers' and therapists' emotional health, and as such offered in-house support and therapy sessions. Being part of a group with my work family, whom I loved dearly, made passing the tissue box and the conversations helpful.

I did not anticipate a positive experience with this breast cancer support group. I worried that if I had to say something, I would be blubbering in waves of sobs, I would not be able to organize my anxieties into cohesive sentences, and the tissue box would be empty. Having Colleen there was going to be my buffer. She knew exactly what to say without looking too upset.

The meeting was held in a small conference room at the Holiday Inn. Colleen scoped out the lobby before we rode the elevator. No bar! Not a good sign.

We walked into the conference room to find twenty women between fifty and seventy years old, in all shapes and sizes, milling about the room in small, chatty clusters. Their voice volumes were set on shrill. Colleen, five years younger than me, was the baby in the room. I found my social worker friend, shook her hand, and introduced Colleen. We were just in time to put our names in a hat for a raffle and begin the group. Unfortunately, the doctor who was scheduled to speak had canceled, but my friend assured us that we would have an informative session anyway.

We sat in a circle. No one looked ill, weak, sad, or sallow. A few wigs needed to be adjusted, and I also noticed an overdo of makeup on a few others, but otherwise no one stood out as being a cancer patient. Colleen nudged close to me. A round woman in a blindingly pink tunic and short, dark, wispy hair immediately began the conversation. It seemed that the women knew each other very well. They spoke freely, interjected, and affirmed each other's feelings. Colleen and I sat back, amazed at the pace of speech, emotion, whining, and belly laughing. The round woman in the pink tunic monopolized the session with her laments about weight gain, low libido, and hammer toes, all of which made exercising difficult and painful. I wondered if she had exercised before cancer. Unfortunately, we did learn about how high her libido was before cancer.

After forty-five minutes, it was time for a break.

"Maybe this is our chance to hightail it outta here," Colleen whispered.

Just as I was about to make excuses to our hostess, excitement bubbled from the corner of the room. A name was pulled from the hat.

"Colleen Hof-mister!" So much for our getaway plan. We sat quietly for an additional hour. Colleen held the gift bag on her lap. It contained a Pepto Bismol–pink water bottle and a discount membership to a gym somewhere on the north shore.

Driving home I asked Colleen, "When was the last time you were in a gym?"

"High school," she replied.

I finally bought a pocket-sized date book to keep medical, work, and home appointments from colliding with each other. A preliminary physical at Memorial Sloan Kettering gave me the green light to the upcoming treatment. This intense anxiety had an upside: The scale confirmed a twenty-five-pound weight loss since February. My appetite had detoured from my usual stress-eating patterns; I had little interest in food beyond a few bites at each meal. There were lots of leftovers for Matt's lunch these days.

I spoke with my friend Dr. Pam Kurey, an OB-GYN physician who lived and practiced outside of Philadelphia. She assured me that the CMF protocol was the safest and most effective avenue for my type of cancer.

"You should do very well, Ann," she said, "but you will need to learn to pace yourself."

Having a plan made the days better. I had a timeline, a chemo cocktail, and expectations to search and learn. While on the phone at work, I stretched my right arm up to reach over my left shoulder blade and pumped my fingers. I was still numb along the underside of my arm, and occasionally my fingertips tingled sharply. The nerves were healing—a good sign.

chapter sixteen

Reunion

Renee flew in with her family from Chicago. They were staying with her folks in Queens for Passover. She borrowed her father's car to drive out to the island for a visit. We had not seen each other in over a year.

Renee and I had been friends since our Buffalo State College days. How I got to Buffalo State College and met my dear friend was serendipitous.

Although my parents encouraged their daughters to go to college, I was expected to choose a practical and family-friendly career in either nursing, teaching, or engineering (engineering only because my dad strived to boast that one of his children had followed in his footsteps). Staying within commuting distance was another variable to adhere to. Being the oldest, I had to set the example. This was a tall order for a fair student who just wanted to be a writer, despite my poor spelling skills and slow reading fluency (an inherited form of dyslexia, I later learned). My tendency to faint at the sight of blood (another trait several relatives shared), and nonexistent aptitude or interest in numbers or design nixed any hope for nursing or engineering. A career in education was my only choice.

Unbeknownst to my parents, I conducted some research. I longed for a live-away-from-home college experience, even though nice Italian girls did not live away from home until they were married to nice, preferably Italian, boys. I sent away for education career information and cross-referenced the training programs with state colleges that were not on Long Island, and eventually targeted speech pathology. The only state colleges that offered the degree were located upstate. My high school grades and SAT scores were ultimately not strong enough for acceptance, however, so I began my freshman year at Suffolk Community College to boost my prospects.

That fall, Matt left for his freshman year at the University of Buffalo mechanical engineering program. It was a natural fit for him; he had the smarts and innate ability to understand how things worked. By the spring semester, I was accepted into the speech pathology program at Buffalo State College.

Buffalo was very far away—480 miles. My parents found consolation in the fact that Matt would be just across town, so I would not be so alone in such a cold place. They were warming to Matt. He was always polite and easily joined in our family gatherings and outings. Dad enjoyed sharing his passions for fishing and trouble-shooting motorboat problems with Matt. They spent a lot of time getting under and into engines together. The fact that Matt was not Catholic or even a little bit Italian eventually faded from their priorities.

I met Renee at the college orientation for transfer students. It was my first time away from my family and anything familiar. Renee was a Jewish girl from Queens who was just as sheltered as me. She stood as tall as me but was much thinner, with bright blue eyes and long, straight dark hair. I later learned her hair was as thick and curly as mine but she had a way to get it to fall straight and tamed. Mine was always wild, and I never did master big curlers or a hairdryer.

We talked continuously for the three days. She had a friendly demeanor, an infectious laugh, and a steady pace that balanced my frantic rushing and overthinking. We remained roommates for two years. Although distance and life's paths separated us over the years, we always found a way back to each other. No matter how much time had passed, we could pick up the conversation where we last left off. Those kind of friends are precious and few.

Renee and her husband, Sev, packed their two children, Adriana and Michael, in her father's car and drove from Queens all the way east to Remsenburg. I put out cheeses and crackers and snacks and prepped a salad. Renee and I talked all afternoon. We caught up on every relative and friend we had ever known. The children threw the ball for Petie until his coughing cued them to stop and let him sit between them as they petted and cooed over him. Matt toured Sev through the prospective spring garden. We all sat down together for a meal of mussels in white wine sauce and the fluke Matt had caught the day before, fried up crispy and light. Renee and Sev said they'd never seen their children eat fish so heartily.

As Matt gave detailed directions back to Sunrise Highway to Sev and the children settled into the car, Renee and I bear-hugged each other.

"You're still the same strong roomie I always knew. You will be fine," she reassured me.

Friends are an incredible blessing.

chapter seventeen

Easter Recap

I wanted Robyn home for Easter weekend so I bought her a plane ticket, and she was through the front door by nine thirty Friday night. Sara and Hallie arrived earlier. Even though the house had been stripped to pristine nakedness for the sake of staging for strangers, it felt cluttered and noisy. Everyone was home. Perfect.

The girls and I spent most of Saturday morning sipping coffee and nibbling on bagels. I swiftly reviewed the upcoming treatment and the expected side effects. There would be no need to worry. We laughed at the prospect of eating Robyn's brownies. I quickly changed the subject to Petie's poor heart. We talked about Hallie's graduation from New Paltz, her waiting to hear from graduate schools, and a summer job at Fox News in New York City. Sara lamented over juggling a full-time job while trying to find her niche in the freelance art world. She worked long hours—sometimes six to seven days a week—leaving her little time to prepare her fascinating art for shows. Robyn was awaiting word of acceptance to a four-week summer fine art program in Ireland but needed a summer job when she returned in June. She had joined a Relay for Life team, an American Cancer Foundation fundraiser, with her friends in Fredonia. They all had a family member who had been touched by cancer.

I spent the remainder of Saturday grocery shopping and prepping for our traditional artery-clogging Easter breakfast at home and the gravlax I was bringing to Mom's for Easter dinner. The house soon smelled of roasted garlic, dill, and oils. I was so happy to be cooking fragrant foods for my family. Matt spread lawn seeds, desperate for spring to pop. Sara worked on her taxes on the dining room table, and Hallie primped for a date with a local boyfriend. In the cool of the afternoon, Robyn rode her bicycle into Westhampton Beach to hunt for a summer job. Home hummed along normally.

chapter eighteen

Vein Hunts

From: Colleen
To: Antoinette
Date: Tuesday, April 10, 2007 at 10:45 a.m.
Subject: Hi Ann!

Just wanted to let you know that you are in my thoughts and prayers ALL of the time. Hope the treatment goes much better than anticipated and includes a pool boy and tropical drinks afterwards!! XXOO

Colleen

The first treatment was at two forty-five. Matt met me at home in the afternoon so we could drive to Commack together. Dr. Sheren greeted us warmly. She tapped my file and reported that the MammaPrint did not yield any new information. She strongly believed we were on the right path.

Since I'd had lymph nodes removed from my right arm,

my left arm veins were the only option for the IV. Rose Ann, the nurse who worked alongside Dr. Sheren, tied the tourniquet and noted how small and deep the veins were. As she slapped my arm and hand to raise a vein, the familiar tunnel vision, light-headedness, and overall body weakness quietly overtook me. Matt caught me as I faded into a slump.

Rose Ann was immediately sympathetic. "I am so sorry. I didn't mean to hurt you."

"She always faints for blood work and IVs." Matt guided me to lie down on the examination table.

"I'm sorry," I said, pressing tears back. "It doesn't hurt. It's just that I am such a baby."

Another attempt yielded just enough blood for the blood test before the vein rolled the needle out of place and I fainted again.

"This is a vasovagal response," Dr. Sheren said. "We should discuss a mediport." She explained that a port could be surgically placed in my chest for easy access to a major vein with a quick puncture. The line would run from a vein in my neck to the port. All blood work, chemotherapy, and anything else that might need to be administered intravenously could be done through the port. No tourniquet, no vein stick. Once treatment was complete, the mediport could be removed. There would be a small scar.

Matt nodded. I shook my head and shivered at the thought of all that invasion.

"We'll think about it," Matt said.

Dr. Sheren decided to get today's IV inserted in the infusion room, where I could lie in a comfortable lounge chair under a warm blanket.

The sunny infusion room was partitioned with short curved walls into what seemed to be a dozen or so stations. Each station had an oversized recliner, chair, IV pole, television, selection of DVDs and books, and basket of cookies. The whole room buzzed with activity and quiet chatter. Matt and I were directed to a station in front of the nurses' desk. A friendly nurse welcomed us, confirmed my name and birth date, gave me a bottle of water to start sipping, and began the orientation.

The nurse repeated Dr. Sheren's list of possible CMF side effects: nausea, constipation, diarrhea, increased appetite, and decrease of appetite due to possible changes in taste and/or mouth sores. I should expect my periods to cease, my hair to thin out, and my skin to be super-sensitive to the sun. She added that since my immune system would be compromised, I needed to avoid raw fish (no sushi!) and salad bars (there goes lunch), wear gloves when gardening and cleaning, and use a commercial veggie wash to thoroughly wash raw vegetables. In short, I should practice germ-phobic habits.

This protocol may become an issue with my home visits, I thought. *It just may be my excuse to resign from the agency.* Little perks kept cropping up.

The "best" vein-hunter nurse was recruited to the room. She hovered over my left arm, pulled the tourniquet, and placed a warm compress in the crook of my elbow.

"Hm, it's a good thing they called me in," she said to my arm. "These are tiny veins."

"Great, the one part of me that is petite."

She began to gently slap a vein, trying to get it to rise closer to the surface.

"Just ignore me and get it in," I said, covering my eyes with my right arm.

She gently pulled my arm from my eyes and looked in my eyes. "We never ignore any of our patients here. Besides, it's in. You did great."

Matt kissed the top of my head and sat in the nearby chair, relieved. He reached for a cookie pack.

Within minutes the drip was plugged in and the titration speed set, allowing the poison to course through my body. I pressed myself deeper into the recliner, careful not to move my left arm.

Right then and there I felt like a woman with cancer. Here I sat, a tube thrust into my vein, dependent on the miracle of science and compassion of these strangers. I wondered if I would morph into a sad, sick woman in need of attention, whose every body function was public knowledge. Or would this cocktail give me superhuman powers? I'm not sure what powers could be possible. Maybe the power of mystery and marvel?

I looked around at my new community. A woman across from my station sat sallow and still in her chair. Her head was perfectly round, with a light fuzz orbiting the top. A nest of auburn waves sat on her lap. The man behind me did not stop talking to anyone who was within his sight. He asked about a nurse's son's upcoming communion, traded a friendly greeting and high five with an attendant, and commented about a book he was reading to the lady across from me. She was glad he was enjoying it. I couldn't see him, but Matt exchanged a friendly nod with him then quickly distracted himself by flipping through a magazine.

An older lady wearing a pink-and-yellow turban was escorted to the station in front of me. She was accompanied by her daughter, I assumed, who carried a pink tote bag with a newspaper and knitting needles packed on the top. I made a mental note to remember a small crochet project for next time, although I wasn't sure if I could crochet without moving my left arm. The two women quickly settled in, and within a few minutes her chemo cocktail was dripping into her body.

Nurse Master Vein Hunter came back into my station with a warm blanket. "You're cold," she said. "The drugs will bring down your body temperature a bit."

I hadn't even realized I was shivering. "Thank you."

"You see the lady in front of you?" the nurse asked. "She has a mediport. It makes chemo days so much easier for her. There's no tourniquet, no missed sticks—although I never miss." She winked at me.

Matt and I turned toward the lady. Her gray eyes looked up at us. She had a long, thin face, but the dab of rouge, penciled eyebrows, and pink lipstick she wore brightened her smile. She pulled down the collar of her blouse to show where the IV was inserted and taped on her chest.

"No big deal," she called over to me. Her daughter handed the knitting to her. Both arms and hands moved freely.

"That may be much better than battling your arm every three weeks," Matt said.

I nodded, but the thought of a lump sticking out of my chest made me shiver under the warm blanket. Matt opened another cookie pack and read the brochure.

After two hours, the final drug had to be administered.

Nurse Master Vein Hunter straddled a rolling stool and pulled a stainless steel tray next to me.

"Last push!" she announced. "How are you feeling?"

I had to admit, I felt pretty good. I think I dozed off for a while, and I didn't feel nauseous, frantic, or too tired. Maybe I could say I felt "well rested." The nurse swabbed and inserted a hypodermic vial into the IV.

"This medicine is thick, so I have to push it in slowly." She fussed with the site as she carefully plunged. I could feel a throb throughout my arm and wrist, and my fingers stung hot.

"Sorry, sorry, I will go slower. Try not to move," she repeated as I winced.

Twenty slow minutes later, she pulled the tube out and sat back. "Honey, your small, rolly veins mean a slow drip and push. I'm not sure if this vein can take eight treatments of this. A port would be so much more comfortable for you. You would get done faster, and once this is over, you can have it removed."

I blew out a big sigh to calm down from this push.

"Okay, sign me up."

~

From: Antoinette
To: My Everyone
Date: Tuesday, April 10, 2007 at 7:20 p.m.
Subject: An update

One down, seven to go. First day of treatment proved that although I am a big girl, I have petite veins that take forever to let in a drip. Getting blood drawn and an IV started was the

worst part, and there was always the threat that my veins would roll and spit the damn thing out. Who knew they had a mind of their own? I am scheduled to have a mediport placed in a few weeks. Everything can be done through this port without tourniquets or needle sticks. It is the lesser of the two nastys. In the meantime, the CMF cocktail was OK. I felt fine, got up easily enough, and left with no problems. Matt and I had a late lunch/early dinner at the pizza shop (eggplant parmesan heals all wounds according to me), and here I am, writing the update.
I got the dos and don'ts while going through the procedure. Gloves while gardening (I do that already), alcohol infrequently (sigh—I continue to be the designated driver), and an uptick in germ management. That last one is going to be a challenge when I visit my snotty nose babies. Another big challenge is not eating raw vegetables. Snacking on pea pods and grape tomatoes from the garden is out! No berries, like my favorite strawberries, since there are too many nooks and crannies for germs to hide in.

I plan to be OK. I have a script for nausea, but reading the side effects is scary. I will have to gauge how bad nausea can be. So that's the scoop. I'm fine. Summer is near—the best medicine.

Thank you all again and again. Your prayers, thoughts, and positive energies are coming through.

Hug everyone you know.
Antoinette

chapter nineteen

Keeping God Real

I was feeling pretty good, not too tired. I went to work for the rest of the week. I did notice I could not eat my usual volumes. I was not going to risk a bout of vomiting, so I kept sipping water and eating little bits at a time. I did immediately discover that sweets tasted like tin. The smell of chocolate triggered a metal taste in my mouth and a roll of nausea. Robyn's brownies sat in the freezer.

Matt's sister Carla asked us to come for dinner on Friday night. She and her mother, Helga, lived in front of the Sayville lot Matt and I had bought to build our new house—which was beginning to seem like it might never happen, since there had been barely a trickle of interested buyers willing to even look at our Remsenburg house.

Matt and his two sisters grew up in the cozy cape when the street was unpaved and children played outdoors until dusk. But time marched forward on Dewey Street, just like every other street, bringing pavement, a few new houses, home extensions, and family turnover. The only constant was the Martins' little red house at the end of the street. My mother-in-law, widowed almost twenty years, stoically remained. Recently her health had been dramatically deteriorating, forcing her into reluctant retirement as a head nurse in a doctor's office. She was losing her Teutonic strength and, worse yet, her sharp mind.

Carla lived with Helga and had taken over the care and attention of the yard, the household, and her mother with incredible skill and energy. If we could build the house in the back lot, we would be more helpful to Helga and Carla as things progressed and also be close by when Carla would be alone.

Matt picked up a bottle of scotch Helga appreciated. We brought Petie, who always enjoyed a car ride and curling up next to Helga. Carla grilled steaks and somehow roasted beets and fennel to gourmet perfection.

As we sat down together, Carla offered grace.

"Thank you, Lord, for the food we are about to eat. We just ask you to pay attention. Keep Antoinette well and strong as she goes through this treatment."

"Amen," Helga said.

"Amen," I echoed.

"I'm not thanking God for anything," Matt said. "I'm too angry."

Helga nodded in agreement and took a sip of her scotch.

Driving home, I told Matt that I would not believe that this cancer was God's fault. I was a bit surprised to find myself saying this out loud. My Catholic conscience usually kept me on guard for the slightest infractions. I was usually on high alert, convinced that any ill wishes or slothful procrastinations could be grounds for divine punishment—and, being the "good girl," managed my own penance before God could take notice. If God had anything to do with this cancer, I thought, perhaps it was to snap me out of my monotonous comfort zone and prove myself to be braver than I could ever dream.

"Cancer is a big attention getter," I said. "But I would have been just as attentive with a talking burning bush. Just saying."

Matt smiled. "I can still be angry." He grinned wider. "And I will never be thankful for beets."

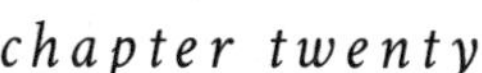

chapter twenty

I'm Fine?!

I could not stay awake. I ached for a horizontal position. A fog hovered over me, muddling my memory and thinking. Reading became a chore. The day prior, I had untangled clumps of hair from my fingers. A pyramid of hair sat on my dresser.

"It's not that much," I reasoned as I threw it away.

To make the days even more difficult, Petie's echocardiogram confirmed a significant heart murmur. His oversized heart displaced his trachea and caused him to hack like a two-pack-a-day smoker. I told him he had better respond to his meds. I had no time for this.

Poor Petie looked so sad when he could not find any of his tennis balls I had to hide. Willow ignored his pleading eyes and gently swatted his nose. Telling a Jack Russell terrier not to play is a torturous prescription.

I had the foresight to put a pork roast in the Crock-Pot on Wednesday morning. When I got home from work, Petie and I trudged up the stairs. I kicked off my shoes and promised him just a half-hour nap. He happily jumped on the bed and nuzzled next to me.

Matt called an hour later. I groggily acknowledged that he was on his way home, then fell back asleep.

He shook me awake at seven thirty. Dinner was ready and the table was set. I managed to get downstairs, eat a few bites, and then slog back up to bed. I was in pajamas and under the covers by eight thirty.

This had better not be me for the next six months, I thought. I just couldn't afford not to work. My salary was what got us over the hump. Besides, the house had to be kept tidy and ready for a walk-through. No one wants to see a fat middle-aged woman sleeping off chemo side effects when they come to look at their potential future home.

Ten days after the chemotherapy treatment, the fog finally lifted. I could read the newspaper and remember what I read. I could smell the coffee from the break room, and I could move. I bounced from my desk to the filing room, made an excuse to get something from my car, then skipped back to my desk. I stood up and paced while speaking on the phone. I put in a full day, came home, and did not head to my bed for a nap. I just kept moving.

I prepared a fabulous meal—osso buco, something I had never cooked before. It needed to roast for many hours, giving me plenty of time to whip up a side of vegetables and a salad, and to vacuum the house. Matt brought home a bottle of wine. A good day.

I cleaned the house early on Saturday morning. A potential buyer came in with the realtor before lunch, took five minutes to walk through the house and yard, and then left. No interest or offer.

A headache grabbed me early in afternoon, forcing me to sit down. It passed within an hour, and I was soon raking leaves from the flower beds and planting peas and lettuce. For dinner, I cooked a manly meatloaf—Matt's favorite.

On Sunday, I walked two miles to the end of Club Lane. The bay glistened in the promising spring sunshine. A deep breath of salt air revived all energies and hope. Matt buffed the boat, and I finished the laundry and caught up on e-mail.

I can do this, I thought.

Matt finished his boat chores early, so we were able to get to Mom and Dad's for Sunday dinner. I brought marinated veggies.

I have to get work's paper flurry under control and keep focused in organizing plans, I thought as we drove home later that evening. *Keep moving, keep planning. I cannot fit in feeling awful.*

A long, sloppy meltdown was triggered by a neighbor who just happened to be a local realtor we had not contracted. I literally ran into her at the post office. Cozy Remsenburg did not offer postal delivery service, so the post office was a place to meet neighbors on an almost daily basis unless you scheduled postal pickups at off times. Over the years, I had mastered the routines depending upon my social moods.

The neighbor asked about our house sale progress. She knew it sucked. She exclaimed how great I looked (thirty-pound weight loss since January).

I was dressed in my frumpy yard clothes, hoping not to bump into anyone.

"You look so young and wonderful," she said.

I did not want to tell her about the cancer. The hamlet's ears were pricked for the most minuscule of gossip. The school board had not yet met to approve my position, and I was not about to jeopardize that opportunity with any unnecessary information. As the neighbor rattled on, I smiled politely. All I could think was that I was in the middle of fighting this insidious disease and looking better than ever! I understood that people who knew what was going on would compliment for encouragement and politeness's sake. It just hurt coming from someone who was not in the know and walked away thinking she'd paid me the ultimate compliment.

I cried through the remainder of the afternoon, feeling very sorry for myself. Perhaps I was crazy. I wondered if chemo caused mental illness. Matt came home to a puddle of a wife. He made me a tall gin and tonic with the extra limes I liked and cooked pork chops in garlic sauce with broccoli rabe. It smelled delicious, but I could only manage a few bites. My mood became more melancholy when a fistful of hair easily sloughed off my head in the shower.

chapter twenty-one

Everyone's Got Something

Colleen came home from oophorectomy and claimed a chipper attitude. I was so glad to hear she'd gotten kid-glove attention at the hospital where her mom had worked.

I wrote a letter to Terry G. on one of my favorite beach cards. Terry was one of my beach bum friends, a woman who rivaled Matt in surf cast fishing. She collected shells and beach glass with the excitement and awe of a child and epitomized genuine friendship and grace. Leukemia had grabbed her that winter. We had spoken earlier in the week. She was in an isolation room. Her immune system was being obliterated and, in a month, would hopefully be rebooted back to health. It sounded awful and lonely. But Terry was her typical optimistic self. I wrote that Matt and I would happily help get her beach house on Davis Park ready for her homecoming.

From: Barbara
To: Antoinette
Date: Tuesday, May 1, 2007 at 11:34 a.m.
Subject: Hey, how's it going?

Are you feeling OK? Hanging in? I will be coming up for Memorial Weekend. Angie is taking a train from Washington on Wednesday. Brianna and I will drive in on Friday night or early Saturday morning. Will we be celebrating Hallie's graduation and going to the beach? I am so looking forward to the end of the school year. I do need to tutor during the summer, though.

A bit of drama to share . . . I met someone on a dating site. I know, I know. I have been careful, met him in a public restaurant. He is a patent lawyer, and is also a single parent with teenagers (3), likes music, traveling, beaching, too. We'll see. I haven't heard from John in a long while. So now you are tuned in to my soap opera. Think of it as a distraction. Love you. See you soon!

Barbara

~

From: Antoinette
To: Barbara
Date: Tuesday, May 1, 2007 at 7:45 p.m.
Subject: Hey, how's it going?

WOW, you are living an As the World Turns life. I understand you need to meet people, and you have been through a lot and deserve "a life." Just be careful!! You should not be going on these "dates" by yourself.

The port surgery is tomorrow, chemo on Thursday, and I am going to try yoga on Friday. I'm not sure yoga is for me. If I am going to spend an hour and a half on self-improvement, I need a puddle of sweat to prove I did something. We'll see if it can calm me down.

Robyn loaded my iPod and decorated an eye mask so I don't have to endure the brightness of the infusion room and cheery people trying to make conversation about their treatment. I don't need new friends right now.

Did you get a referral for an MRI yet? Just do it, Barb. You have young girls to raise and don't need this detour. Diana did it, and she is free and clear. Relief! Can't wait to see you and my nieces. Love you. Be good. Be well!

Hug everyone you know.
Ann

~

From: Barbara
To: Antoinette
Date: Tuesday, May 1, 2007 at 8:33 p.m.
Subject: Hey, how's it going?

Yes, I got the referral. I will make sure I keep the "twins" healthy as well as the rest of me starting with me controlling my weight. I know I need to pay attention to myself and eat salad! I'll keep you in the loop on this new guy. We'll talk soon.

Barbara

Everyone had something; my sisters were no different. With less than four years between myself and my youngest sister (the fourth of five siblings), our sisterhood relationships were a spectrum of ups and downs. We each grew to be women with diverse temperaments, different theories and practices in the nurturing of our families, and, somehow, varying perceptions of our idyllic childhood. In the end, though, we were all emotionally attached, not just by history or blood ties but by a genuine feeling of love and friendship for each other.

My two other sisters, brother, and I remained local, but Barbara had followed her husband's career until they finally settled in a Virginia suburb of Washington, DC. Barbara's nineteen-year marriage had collapsed two years before when her husband basically decided he did not want their life together anymore. She had been left to redefine her role as a parent of two teenage daughters, homemaker, teacher, and now ex-wife. This abrupt change was wrought with false starts and insecurities. I had tried to be the nonjudgmental sister-friend, offering an ear for her to vent to and baby-step advice to navigate the enormity of each challenge. She had always been an exhaustive talker and a fun-seeking person who easily made friends wherever she went. Thankfully, she had a large circle of local friends with local shoulders to cry on. I felt honored that she reached out to me, the reliable older sister.

I worried about my sisters' health as well as the future health of my daughters and nine nieces. Genetic testing revealed no known genetic traits for breast cancer, but many unknown genetic traits had not yet been discovered. My maternal grandmother and mother had both had breast cancer. With that history, I urged my sisters to request a breast MRI. It was difficult for a standard mammogram to see everything in large, dense breasts. Mary and Diana were checked, but Barbara kept stalling, blaming everything that robbed time. I was relieved by her most recent e-mail's report that she was taking proactive steps toward better health. Her love life, however, was another worry.

chapter twenty-two

A Port Story

Wednesday was port placement day. I had been an anxious wreck since deciding to go through with it, despite the doctor's assurance that the surgery was a piece of cake. I couldn't sleep for more than a few hours, couldn't remember anything on my ever-growing lists, couldn't recall if I had talked to Sara or was it Robyn or was it my sister? In the early morning on the day of the surgery, I saw that my shirt needed to be ironed and then couldn't find my sneakers.

"Time to go!" Matt hollered from the front door. We were going to hit rush-hour traffic to the hospital.

"Okay! Okay!" I shouted back. I slipped into loafers and buttoned the cotton shirt with a wrinkled collar.

The vein search and stick was as tough as expected. It took two attempts to get the needle to stay in my arm. The patient nurse confirmed that I was a prime candidate for this procedure.

"It will be so much easier on you. You are going to love it."

I did not think there was any procedure I could love, but I would appreciate being comfortable.

The doctor explained the procedure. He had a confident manner and assured me that the whole thing would be quick and relatively painless. The twilight sedative would leave me very calm. I would only remember him singing his favorite oldies tunes.

The surgery, however, was far from a piece of cake. It turned out that the twilight had an opposite effect on me. Instead of being quiet and calm as the surgeon made an incision in my neck to feed the tube to where the port would lodge in my chest (big YUCK), I was extremely agitated and not unconscious.

"Am I supposed to feel this?" I stammered.

He ordered more medication, hoping it would kick in, and began to sing along to Frankie Valli's "Let's Hang On." The humor soon faded as I began to hyperventilate and felt my whole body wrapped in a cold sweat.

"I can't give you any more medication," the doctor said.

"It might be easier to knock me over the head with a shovel," I suggested through the shivering.

"We can't do that," the nurse said as she put an oxygen cannula into my nose. "But Doctor can work faster and stop singing."

She held my hand through the rest of the surgery. I apologized for squeezing so hard.

I left ambulatory surgery with pressure bandages covering the stitches on my neck and chest that would dissolve, and a tube attached to the embedded port taped and ready to go for the next day's chemo treatment. At home, I crawled into bed with my wounds, both physical and emotional. Petie sighed beside me. The Vicodin the surgeon had prescribed had my head swirling all night. I felt that I was falling out of bed all night.

I woke up exhausted but could not cancel the early intervention morning meeting I had scheduled. It was too important. The young Muslim mother was very anxious over her weak twelve-month-old son who had been born ten weeks premature and showed severe neurological disabilities. I wanted to be sure the family received the services the child needed within the parameters of their culture.

I had met with the mother, child, grandmother, and aunt a few times in their lovely suburban home. The women were well educated and spoke perfect English. Both of the young parents had been born and raised in New York. Although they had adopted many Western customs, their traditions remained strong and needed to be respected. When I first entered their home and removed my shoes, two men, probably the dad and grandfather, stood in the kitchen entry, listening. Muslim men were not permitted to speak to non-Muslim women, and Muslim women were not allowed to speak with non-Muslim men. The county representative had to be switched, and I had to coordinate evaluators and therapists accordingly. There were also specific times in the day that had to be observed.

I had been warned by a few officemates that "these" families were usually demanding and expected special attention and treatment. Instead, I found the women welcoming, sincere, and appreciative of my efforts in getting everything that was needed to help their beautiful child. The baby had long, gorgeous lashes. We joked about how strong his big brown eyes must be to lift such thick, heavy lashes.

The meeting went smoothly. Services were approved, goals written, and the women and I were pleased. I saw the father, a thin beard outlining his long face, peek around the kitchen corner. As I prepared to leave, the mother walked me to the door.

"Are you okay?" she asked.

This was one of the few mothers I had told about the cancer. Because she was new to my caseload, I had given her the option to be assigned to a different coordinator. But she said she felt comfortable with me and, most importantly, trusted me.

"I'm fine," I said. "I had surgery yesterday and I have a treatment this afternoon, so I'm a little sore and anxious. But we had a great meeting for your son! I have the therapists lined up and ready to contact you. It will be a long road, but we have an excellent start."

"Thank you." She lightly hugged me. "My husband and father-in-law thank you as well." She hugged me again. "We will all pray for you."

I was raised Catholic but had not been involved with my parish for most of my adult life. Matt was raised in a Lutheran household. The church was his extended family throughout his childhood. We had tried several Protestant churches. I was always astounded by how easy it was to go from church to church. That was never an option as a Catholic. One attended the neighborhood parish, no questions asked.

Eventually, Matt and I abandoned the dogma of organized religion and church altogether. That did not mean, however, that I had no faith. I truly believed in the existence of an almighty being, God, the loving messages of Jesus Christ, the power of positive energies from the teaching of saints (the ancient as well as those who walk among us), and the awe-inspiring beauty of nature. I was not about to dismiss the extra voices and meditations calling out for my safe and successful passage through this cancer. Now, along with God and Jesus Christ, I had Allah's attention. It was so appreciated, welcomed, and comforting.

My spirits were deflated when I stopped by the office and learned that Marcia from the accounting cubicle had experienced a severe stroke the night before. She had just visited last week, sporting a wig that looked like her red pixie style. She came in with her son to see everyone and catch up on the latest office gossip. Maybe she had really come to say goodbye.

From: Antoinette
To: My Everyone
Date: Thursday, May 3, 2007 at 9:45 p.m.
Subject: Round Two

Two down! I had a second chemo treatment this afternoon, which, after I was given a Percocet for pain from yesterday's surgery, Ativan for general anxiety, and no vein stick thanks to the handy dandy port, all went pretty smoothly and quickly (one and a half hours). The port surgery yesterday was not as smooth. I am learning that when doctors say a procedure is a "piece of cake," it really means it is easy for them and a horror show for me. The sedation didn't work and had me just about jumping out of my skin even with a maximum dose. I felt everything when I was supposed to be calm and pliable. A kind nurse held my hand through it all. I hoped I didn't snap a bone.

I am actually feeling pretty good now. My nurse at Sloan fixed the bandage, making it much more comfortable to move my neck and shoulders. The whole chemo experience was relatively painless. Matt and my mom met me at Sloan to keep me company. I put on the eye mask Robyn painted for me that looked like I was wide awake with heavily mascaraed lashes and glittery green eye shadow. Mom brought her Palm Pilot with an audible e-book. I was lulled into a floating nap (a nice treat in the middle of the day). Matt and I drove home, stopped for a broiled scallops takeout, and here I am, writing to all of you.

My hair is steadily shedding, but I have plenty, so it is not noticeable. My hat order should be arriving any day now. The garden is in: lettuce, broccoli rabe, and sweet peas have sprouted. Matt is diligently watering grass, flowers, and the garden to lure a house buyer. The new gas tank for the boat came yesterday, so he will be spending the weekend installing it and painting the boat bottom. Maybe we will be able to open the pool on Sunday. We are plowing forward, not letting this inconvenience our everyday.

I am hoping this note finds you all well. Take good care of yourselves.

Hug everyone you know.
Antoinette

From: Stefano
To: Antoinette
Date: Friday, May 4, 2007 at 2:45 a.m.
Subject: Round Two

Ciao, Ann. Right now, I am in Rio de Janeiro tanning on the top floor of my hotel on Ipanema beach and sipping an icy capipiroska (I had too many and cannot spell it anymore). They have wireless Internet so I am trying to check my email (because I' m supposed to be working here) while I stare at the curvy, topless, and friendly local beauties.

Wow, what an ordeal you are going through. I cannot possibly imagine all the emotions, but I am sure you have a smile and a joke for everyone, either at home or at the hospital. I think this is truly a sign of your strength, which is so big that you can always afford to lend some of it to people around you. And I don't think there is a better way of doing it than with your beautiful smile.

Baci,
Stefano

From: Dr. Pam
To: Antoinette
Date: Friday, May 4, 2007 at 9:45 p.m.
Subject: Round Two

You are getting through this. It seems when we docs do things all the time, we forget that it is the first time for most of our patients. I wish I could have been there for the port to hold your hand and tell them to give you better stuff. You will be glad you have that port. Now your blood draws and treatments can be done through that little magic button. You and Colleen remain on our prayer list at church. I enjoy hearing from you and hope you continue to keep us posted. Please keep that great smile and super attitude. We love you, Ann.

Pam

~

From: Gloria
To: Antoinette
Date: Friday, May 4, 2007 at 10:33 p.m.
Subject: Round Two

Ann, so glad you are in good spirits and feeling well. Do you have a nurse at home helping you? You have such a great attitude. If you happen to have enough energy, come to my house and get my garden in order (HAHA). We're praying for you, Ann. Stay well.

Gloria

~

From: Antoinette
To: Gloria
Date: Saturday, May 5, 2007 at 11:45 a.m.
Subject: Round Two

A nurse? Come on, Gloria; you know me better. I am going about my everyday just a bit more tired than usual. I refuse to use up my banked days off for this. Vacation is more important. I could use a housekeeper, cook, grocery and errand

> *shopper, dog walker . . . you know—a wife. I would be glad to come help you with the garden. We have a rototiller, a very fun tool.*

On Friday, I walked into a neighborhood yoga studio. My friend Anne suggested that yoga practice might help relieve some tension and allow me to stretch guarded muscles. Physical grace had never been my strong skill. I surprised myself by being able to hold several beginner poses—but I just could not coordinate my breathing. The mediation part of the session, where I had to lie on the floor and let my mind be one with my breathing, proved especially difficult. My right foot would not stop shaking. A headache crept in, probably due to the incense burning. The instructor encouraged me to return and practice again.

"You must learn to be alone, with yourself, in your own mind," she said.

I am the last person my mind should be alone with, I thought. This might not be the right time to explore yoga.

chapter twenty-three

Death

Thursday, May 10, 2007

Marcia died. After a four-month battle with lung cancer, she is forever gone. She endured a nasty chemo cocktail that did not buy her the time she wanted. She had brand-new grand-twins, children, a sister who had been her lifelong best friend, nieces and nephews, and numerous friends and coworkers—her adjunct family. She was doomed at diagnosis.

The temple was packed. The eulogy was so sad yet celebrated the little lady who lived as a strong, wise, and loving person. She truly enjoyed the humble gifts life dealt her. My heart broke as the simple coffin was led down the aisle and her daughter's sobs echoed, "Mama! Mama!"

Good-bye, Marcia. I was lucky to have known you.

chapter twenty-four

May Days

From: Antoinette
To: My Everyone
Date: Sunday, May 13, 2007 at 8:26 a.m.
Subject: Happy Mother's Day

Happy Mother's Day to all of you sister-mommies. We are so blessed to have such wonderful people to nurture. We sweat, worry, bleed, cry, advise, laugh, dance, and celebrate over our cherubs. It is, by far, the most exhausting yet most rewarding job. And they are damn lucky to have us as their mothers. Enjoy the beautiful day.

Hug everyone you know.
Ann

The port looked like an alien poking through my chest—UGLY! It was not as comfortable as the sales pitch promised. I could not sleep on my left side. I became a guarded hugger. It felt too big. Could this space in my chest be another petite body part? It did, however, work well for the treatment. Knowing that it would come out as soon as I was through with all this cancer crap balanced the discomfort.

I found that this chemo cocktail was not so bad. For a few days after the treatment I trudged through my workdays, marathon sleeping and being acutely aware of how food was making me feel, but after that I did not feel overly tired or too nauseous. Even my period came right on time. The constipation was solved with two to three glasses of Metamucil each day. I discovered that if I kept a reasonable schedule and pace at work and took a forty-five-minute couch nap instead of burying myself under the comforter and pillows on my bed as soon as I arrived home, I could manage my daily to-do list much more efficiently. I missed chocolate, though. The smell of it still triggered a metallic taste in my mouth and a tsunami wave of nausea.

May burst with events requiring my master-mom coordinator skills. Matt and I spent Mother's Day weekend driving nine hours to Fredonia, collecting Robyn and her stuff into the minivan, and leaving Fredonia for what we thought might be forever. Robyn had successfully applied for transfer to the University of Buffalo (sixty miles northeast of Fredonia) in hopes that the environmental science and art programs might be a better fit. She had also been accepted to a SUNY summer abroad fine art program in Dingle, Ireland. For four weeks, she was going to paint pastures and sea landscapes.

There was so much to prepare before she left in two weeks. As we drove down Route 81, I rattled out the lists of supplies and shopping we needed to do. Robyn insisted that one change of underwear, an extra T-shirt, and her Tyvek sandals would suffice. It was extremely frustrating to impress upon her the importance of being prepared for nasty weather and rocky terrain, and that packing a few shirts, a sweatshirt, and *several* panties was absolutely necessary. It was a long nine-hour drive back home.

Hallie's graduation from SUNY New Paltz was the following weekend. New Paltz was less than a three-hour drive—a rather lovely ride along the scenic Hudson River. Getting off Long Island took strategic planning, between the congested expressway, bridge delays, and cantankerous New York drivers. I had arranged for hotel rooms and dinner reservations for the night before graduation the previous October, knowing it would be impossible once the date approached.

Hallie had to move out of her hovel apartment after the graduation ceremony. Unlike Robyn, my middle daughter had an enormous amount of stuff and books she could not bear to leave behind. We were going to need as many cars as possible. Matt and I drove the minivan with Sara and Robyn. My parents left in their car. We started from Remsenburg by eleven fifteen in the morning and checked into the hotel two hours and forty-seven minutes later—our best time yet.

Matt and Sara went into town to meet Hallie, and Robyn found a nearby trail to hike. My parents were not expected for a few hours, so I took a nap.

Three hours later, everyone tumbled into my room. Dad was surprised to see that I was just waking up.

"You're sleeping!" he said. "Are you sick? Maybe this is too much for you."

"I'm up, Dad," I said, stretching. "I'm fine."

"But you never sleep during the day."

"And I've never had chemo, either."

Rain threatened graduation day. Gray clouds let out a light drizzle, dampening the outdoor seats. Oddly, there was no plan B for inclement weather. No matter, by the time the graduates marched in, the sun shone bright and hot.

My family stood up to watch Hallie walk for her well-deserved diploma, honor tassel hanging from her robe. I held my mother's hand as she stood on tiptoes, straining her neck to see above the crowd. I felt her strength. She never let obstacles get in her way. What an amazing gift to have this woman as my mother and strong role model.

Despite our distance from the stage, we saw my girl's infectious smile when her full name, Hallie Diane Martin, was called.

During the afternoon reception, we met Hallie's professors, who genuinely gushed over her skills and acceptance to the journalism program at Northwestern University Medill College in Chicago. What a proud day.

The Saturday of Memorial Day weekend was penned in the calendar to celebrate Hallie's graduation at home. I already had lists of dishes to prepare and groceries to buy hanging on the refrigerator. Lots to do, lots to plan—loved it.

chapter twenty-five

Growing Pains

I packed a tote bag with my crochet project, a case folder to maybe work on, a book, and my glittery eye mask. After the treatment, I planned to shop at the nearby Costco for the weekend's bulk party supplies and a few things for Robyn's Ireland trip.

I had barely put my bag down in the waiting room when my name was called. A deep breath, a stab to the port, and within a minute blood was being drawn and the IV line placed. Nurse Rose Ann reviewed symptoms. I reported that I was fine and joked that perhaps they hadn't given me the full hit last time since I was so pathetic after the port surgery.

Dr. Sheren strolled in with her warm smile. "Your white blood count is too low for chemotherapy today," she said.

"No chemo?" I'd never imagined being disappointed in not having chemotherapy.

Dr. Sheren explained that it was too dangerous, even though it was borderline. I also had a mouth sore and a cough. While the chemotherapy attacked the cancer cells, it also poisoned healthy cells, including infection-fighting white blood cells. She prescribed an injection of Neulasta to stimulate my bone marrow to produce more white blood cells. Another injection was scheduled for two days later.

"We'll see how you feel on Thursday," said the doctor.

"I feel fine now," I said.

The nurse removed the IV line from the port and then administered a shot in my arm. I never had problems with shots since they did not involve veins. I picked up my bag and headed for home to "rest."

~

From: Antoinette
To: My Everyone
Date: Tuesday, May 22, 2007 at 5:43 p.m.
Subject: Sidetrack

I was supposed to have chemo today, but my white blood cell count was too low, even though I felt fine. I got two shots of Neulasta to boost the counts. Hopefully it will work, and I can get back on track with the chemotherapy on Thursday. The shot is supposed to get the bone marrow working to make more white blood cells. I will need another shot the day after chemo to keep the bone marrow producing. I can't believe that I am so disappointed in not getting chemo today . . . BLAH.

Hug everyone you know.
Antoinette

~

From: Sara
To: Antoinette
Date: Tuesday, May 22, 2007 at 10:02 p.m.
Subject: Sidetrack

Oh, Mom, you're like chemo hard core. I am working on getting my health checked out, just like you nagged. I had my physical today and got a tetanus shot. I will upload the graduation pictures later tonight. I will see you on Saturday for the party. Can someone pick me up at the Speonk station?

Sara

~

I was not fine during the night. My legs and arms ached, making any position uncomfortable within minutes. Waves of nausea kept me worried I might vomit. Smells and tastes triggered metallic sensations. I sipped ice water and plain tea. I worried that this sidebar would drag out the treatment protocol. I wanted this chemo trip to be done and over in time to start my new position at Remsenburg-Speonk. It was a long night.

I went back to Memorial Sloan Kettering by myself on Wednesday afternoon for the Neulasta shot and confirmed the chemo appointment for Thursday afternoon. My bones ached. I felt like I was growing all day and night. I took half a Percocet Wednesday night to help bring on some much needed sleep.

Thursday's blood work reported normal white blood count levels. The Neulasta shots had worked. I sat in the infusion lounge chair hooked up to the CMF drip, relieved to be there. Crazy!

I went back for a long-lasting hit of Neulasta on Friday. I was back on schedule.

Keeping white blood cell counts within normal limits during chemotherapy came with a price. I officially felt awful. Moving hurt. Staying still hurt more. Bed, couches, and chairs could not offer any respite from the bone agony and fatigue. All food smells volleyed nausea, threatening to purge my already empty stomach.

I had to postpone the graduation party for a couple of weeks. The exhaustion and pain won out. Damn it! Robyn would be in Ireland, but everyone else juggled their schedules to make it work and offered to bring their specialties.

"No problem, Ann," Barbara said over the phone. "I can stay home this weekend and drive up for the party in two weeks. I'm bringing my famous fruit salad."

I love my family.

I was weepy, and the fatigue from the pain kept me slow and frustrated. The doctor and nurses warned that I would be feeling exceptionally achy with the three shots and chemo session, but it should dissipate. I was still sulking over postponing the party.

Friends came to the rescue. Dan and Coll Kovarick and Chris and Fluke Flaherty came over with their young children to spend Saturday poolside. They brought delicious rubbed meats and fabulous side dishes. The kids splashed and played between the chilly pool and bubbly hot tub. Everyone helped with the cleanup.

On Sunday, Nick and Pam invited Matt and me to come to their Davis Park beach house and stay over for Memorial Day Monday. Davis Park is a small summer community on the eastern portion of Fire Island—a barrier island that protects a thirty-two-mile stretch of Long Island's Suffolk County. It's accessible only by the Patchogue ferry or private boats. The little community was founded after World War II by local mainlanders and remained simple, with just one harbor store, one restaurant with a bar, and boardwalks as street addresses. Wagons were the only vehicles.

Nick and Pam's house overlooked the Great South Bay, three hundred yards from the ocean—perfectly situated for sunset views. It was an old goat barn Pam's grandfather had floated across the bay and "thrown up" on the shore. Years of improvements had shaped it into a cozy beach house.

Through the years, we had been frequent guests. We often rode our boat over to spend the day or weekend. For several seasons, Matt and I were able to rent out our Remsenburg home, located in the "mouth of the elite Hamptons," which allowed us to rent a Davis Park beach house all summer. Matt commuted to work on the mainland daily while the girls and I clammed with our feet, sailed the Sunfish, fished for snappers, caught crabs from the docks with a chicken leg tied to a string, collected shells and beach glass, and dove in and out of the ocean waves. We filled our nights hunting fireflies and toads, grilling dinner, and roasting marshmallows. We painted shells on rainy days. We read books. No one missed the television. Our skin glowed in healthy bronze tones, our hair blew out of hats and clips, stiff from the salty air and water. Our best family portraits were of us all on the beach, windblown and salty in oversized tank shirts and sun-beaten bathing suits.

For over twenty-five years, the Martins had been regulars in Davis Park. I believed the beach was the best and safest place on Earth to let children run and play with pure freedom. I also believed that this beach had much-needed healing properties no pharmaceutical company could duplicate.

Sunday was warm with a light sea breeze. Our twenty-five-foot Pro-Line motorboat hummed through Moriches Bay channel and into the Great South Bay. We spent a relaxing day on Nick and Pam's beautiful deck overlooking a tranquil bay. At night, I was lulled to sleep with the sound of the ocean complementing the ordered rest.

chapter twenty-six

June! It's June!!

Robyn left for Ireland Friday night, called the following morning to report her safe arrival in Dingle, and claimed she had no time to talk. I hoped to hear a little more about the living quarters, roommates, meals, and schedules, but that was Robyn—a minimalist in conversation as well as packing.

Hallie began working at Fox News as a crawl writer, joining the throngs of commuters waiting for trains to bring them to and from New York City. She was originally hired full-time, but her hours were cut to three days a week when she revealed her graduate school plans in Chicago. Luckily, she was able to line up young clients for private swimming lessons. Hallie spent her downtime on craigslist searching for a Chicago apartment and roommates. She also found time to practice with the Long Island Roller Rebels as Candee Catastrophe. I sighed a lot.

The Remsenburg-Speonk school board approved my position! I organized my paperwork and made lists of loose ends to tuck in before I gave the agency notice the following week. A new coordinator had recently been hired, and she had a very light caseload, so I didn't have to feel so guilty about leaving. Meanwhile, my good friend arranged for me to work as a part-time speech therapist for a local summer school program. Everything was falling into place.

About five days after treatment, that chemo fog lifted and my familiar restless energy flooded into my day. Fellow cancer buddies complained of a slow wit, sore muscles, and muddled motivation. Conversely, I buzzed along all day, leaving Post-it notes on eye-level vertical surfaces and scheming for the next day. I abandoned my forty-five-minute couch nap, rationalizing there was no time to fit it in. The "growing pains" flared up when I finally got into bed at night, but Tylenol worked well enough to get me through to morning. I felt fine, really.

chapter twenty-seven

Epidemic

From: Dr. Pam Kurey
To: Antoinette
Date: Tuesday, June 5, 2007 at 7:21 a.m.
Subject: Me too

It was good to talk to you last night. I am scared, Ann. I don't scare easily, but the unknown and whether I will be cured or not leaves me numb. I will keep you posted. Keep me in your prayers. You are in mine.

Pam

What the #@!*? Dr. Pam had breast cancer, too! I felt sick and incredibly sad over the news. We talked on a Monday night, and Dr. Pam, usually confident and optimistic, retold her discovery of a lump and overnight transition from doctor to patient status. I heard fear in her voice. She was a year younger than me and knew firsthand the statistics and risks. She had three young children, ages four to eleven. Her husband, Greg, was genuinely frightened as well. I hoped I offered her words of courage, a bit of experienced wisdom. We shared a short cry. Dr. Pam would have scans and probably a surgery scheduled by the end of the week.

From: Dr. Pam
To: Antoinette
Date: Wednesday, June 6, 2007 at 6:54 p.m.
Subject: Update

Just got back from my bone scan—negative. Chest x-ray—negative. Blood work—negative. All good. My MRI shows a funny spot in my other breast, so I am off to have an MRI-guided biopsy tomorrow. UGH! I'll let you know. I am glad I have you. I talked to our friend Pam B today. It was very hard to tell my childhood friend. Did you cry suddenly for no reason?

Pam

From: Antoinette
To: Dr. Pam
Date: Wednesday, June 6, 2007 at 7:44 p.m.
Subject: Update

I was a constant puddle, and can still cry for what seems to be no reason and every reason possible. Thank God for my Matt, my girls, and an insanely busy schedule. Gin helps, too. There is no shame in crying. You have every right to cry! Just let it out, dry your tears, and keep moving forward.

Ann

Cancer was all around me. Two women I had worked with years earlier found out about my plight and offered their support. They were both about one year out of breast cancer treatment. Janet, an active and very skilled physical therapist, had had a lumpectomy and underwent an aggressive chemotherapy and radiation protocol, leaving her weak and hairless. She'd returned to her gym and maintained a regular workout schedule to ward off depression and build strength. Sherry, a fellow speech therapist who had undergone a unilateral mastectomy, chemotherapy, and radiation, offered tips and tricks to ward off nausea and port discomfort. They were added to my e-mail list.

My beach community of friends had been reaching out to each other as well. It had been a very rough winter, healthwise. Terry was battling leukemia, Colleen and I had been diagnosed with breast cancer, and now Dr. Pam was scheduled for a lumpectomy and node dissection. I also learned that another very young woman on our Pepperidge Walk boardwalk had arrived on the beach with a scarf covering her bare head, her eyelashes and eyebrows absent. Lisa began aggressive chemotherapy for her breast cancer after a unilateral mastectomy just before her fortieth birthday.

How could this be happening? Was cancer some kind perverted rite of passage? It was not just about each individual woman. This disease impacted families, children of all ages, spouses, parents, dear friends, and coworkers. Cancer did not inflict havoc in a vacuum, alone and private. It cruelly teased and frightened us, our families, and friends, while challenging our bodies to defy its advances and defeat it. Right now my friends and I were in good hands, but I tried not to think of who was next.

chapter twenty-eight

NPR Essay

I liked to listen to NPR radio programs. *This I Believe,* a program that invites the public to share the beliefs they practice in their daily lives, aired while I drove to work. I thought of submitting an essay that reflected my current beliefs:

I Believe in Faking It

> *I believe in faking it as I journey through breast cancer treatment. Although my prognosis is positive, I still need to muddle through chemotherapy and, soon after, radiation therapy. I juggle my home and work routines so gaps are not noticeable—as if I have always had time to fit doctor appointments, infusion sessions, and nausea into my day. It takes a lot of planning and preparation, which is a major feat with a chemo brain and poisoned body. I paste a smile on my face and reassure My Everyone that I am fine. The façade keeps those around me calm and superficially convinces me that I am really okay.*

But in reality, the positive attitudes fade away when my body revolts, nightmares are recalled in a wakened state, and thoughts are left to their own ramble. I am very frightened. Questions I dare not give voice to loop through my head. What if this cancer cannot be beaten down? What if I become debilitated and sick for the rest of my life? What if I am robbed of life prematurely? I imagine wasting away while my daughters navigate through their young adulthood without me. I shake at the image of not being part of weddings, unknown to grandchildren, and missing life adventures that lay ahead. Pain would define my legacy. Happier memories would have to be conjured from faded photographs that never got dated, signed, or organized. Who is going to do that now? I am deeply afraid that once an absent memory, I will be replaced. My husband will find a new wife; my daughters will adopt a new mother. Although terrified of that outcome, I am ANGRY that it should be that way if the worst happens.

Anger is another reality. I am so mad at myself for not taking better care of the only body I have and that it betrayed me into believing that I was fine. I am furious that this disease scares my husband and daughters. They have to live with me and watch me go through the protocols. I am livid that cancer surrounds every aspect of life and infects so many lives. This is not supposed to happen!

But crying and ranting will not make cancer go away any faster. Negotiating ignorance and a simpler protocol only flirts with recurrence and extends the horror show. If I show my true anxieties, I risk paralyzing myself further, digging into an abyss and surrendering. Pretending all is well, dragging myself through the day with a smile, and

> *repeating that I am fine keeps the beast at bay. I was never an adequate actress or a gifted liar, but I am rather skilled at believing what I want to believe.*
>
> *I believe I will fare through treatment with minor injury. I believe I will be well for a very long time. I believe I can fake it. This I believe.*

I did not submit this hasty essay. If it were accepted and aired, I feared it might jinx my "good attitude" strategy. Right now, that was the only strategy in my pocket.

chapter twenty-nine

Time for a Party

A beautiful warm day with clear skies showed up for the graduation party. Fifty or so relations and friends came to celebrate Hallie. Everyone brought a dish, and I had meats marinating and platters and bowls lined up ready to be filled. The kids splashed and played in the pool. Matt happily grilled. Mom, sisters, and aunts helped me keep the serving table bursting with food and the kitchen sink clear. My dad, uncles, and cousins played bocce in the side yard where they measured close winners by foot paces and toe length. Even Helga enjoyed the day with us.

The realtor walked into the backyard with prospective buyers during Hallie's graduation party. He apologized for the drop-in and asked if he could show the house. I warned them of the lived-in look of the rooms, with damp towels strewn on furniture, a cluttered kitchen counter, and bakery boxes holding cakes, pies, and cookies scattered on the dining room table and on top of the piano. I knew that Robyn's and my bedroom were tidy. I hoped Sara and Hallie had at least picked up their underwear and wiped away sprays of toothpaste from their bathroom mirror and sink.

"It's a livable mess that makes it a home," I quipped. The buyers were not amused. They were a tall and lean couple dressed in matching chino slacks, light-blue oxford shirts, and large Ray-Ban sunglasses. They could have passed as twins with their whitened teeth and dark hair slicked back into neat ponytails. The only thing differentiating them was that the woman wore a blue silk scarf tied to the base of her ponytail.

The realtor began his rattle about the spaciousness and natural light as he guided them into the house. They completed the house tour within three minutes and came outside to the patio, where Matt was beating down flames on the grill. They looked over the four-foot cedar slat fence into the chaotic fun going on in the pool yard. Gangly teens chased each other into the pool while loud exclamations resounded over an incredible bocce pitch that had just changed the dynamics of the playoff.

I met them from the other side of the fence. "It's a great house to throw a party," I offered.

The realtor agreed. The couple sneered and perhaps, behind their Ray-Bans, rolled their eyes over the crude prospect. They declined a tour around the pool yard, a drink, or a paper plate of food. No matter—it was a great day.

~

From: Dr. Pam
To: Antoinette
Date: Monday, June 11, 2007 at 3:38 p.m.
Subject: What's happened

Ann—it's me, Greg. I just got back from the hospital. The news is fantastic: no node involvement whatsoever! I simply cannot express to you how relieved I am. It's like a cloud has lifted. Now we wait for a call on the margins. Pam is doing well. She is home and sleeping. Thank you for all of your prayers, support, good vibes, and love. As she had probably discussed with you, she will most likely head back to surgery for a mastectomy (bilateral) later. I just want her to be alive and well for many, many years to come. Lots of love,

Greg

~

From: Antoinette
To: Dr. Pam
Date: Monday, June 11, 2007 at 4:24 p.m.
Subject: What's happened

Greg, when she feels up it, she can call any time. Get some rest. It is hard work being the good man through this. Take good care. Sending kisses.

Hug everyone you know.
Ann

chapter thirty

Not So Easy

I asked my hair stylist to cut the back and sides of my hair closer to my head and shape the top. It was noticeably shorter—even Matt commented on it, and he rarely noticed my haircuts. I justified that summer required quick and easy hair, and besides, my hats fit better.

A day later, I finished my fourth treatment—halfway through chemotherapy now. White blood count was good, so everything was a go. Something went wrong with the port, though. It hurt badly as the poison dripped in. The nurse stopped the titration and pulled the needle out. The port site looked tender and slightly swollen. She prepared to poke around for a rolly arm vein. I moaned. Matt stood up.

Matt usually sat in the visitor's chair once we walked into the infusion room station, situated near me but within arm's reach of the cookie basket. Although attentive through my examinations and procedures, he remained the quiet observer. I reported symptoms and asked the questions. He listened and nodded. But now, with the threat of a vein hunt, I was suddenly speechless, and he pounced into rescue mode. He loomed his six-foot-three self between me and the nurse sitting on the rolling stool and insisted that placing an IV in my arm was not an option. The nurse, who was new to me, insisted it would not be a big deal.

"It is a big deal," he said with increasing volume. "She is not going through this session with an IV in her arm. Try the port again."

Dr. Sheren was called in, a discussion between all four of us ensued, and then the doctor and nurse stepped away for more discussion. Finally, Dr. Sheren returned with her calming smile.

"We'll try the port with a smaller needle," she said. "It may take a little longer but should be more comfortable."

The nurse returned with a fresh prep, carefully placed the needle into the port, and reset the titration. Matt sat back down, relieved. I dug deeper into my chair and pulled my eye mask down. It was better but not painless. I dared not complain.

~

From: Antoinette
To: My Everyone
Date: Wednesday, June 13, 2007 at 7:52 p.m.
Subject: Midway

I had my fourth midway treatment today. It was a near disaster when, after twenty minutes of being plugged in via the port, I felt sharp pains and throbbing. The last two times, the port was absolutely painless, thereby well worth the fact that it looks like a small alien is bursting through my chest. I should have said nothing since the nurse was ready to start searching for an arm vein . . . negating the whole reason for the port. Matt came to the rescue and insisted that vein stabbing was not happening. After some back and forth (Matt growing loudly insistent), my doctor came in and suggested a different size needle to place in the port. Ativan for anxiety dripped through first, and I nodded off with Robyn's kooky eye mask and iPod on. I think Matt could have used the same.

I will now be getting the day-after-chemo injection, Neulasta, to keep those white blood cells in good number to fight off infections. Last month, I had the expected bone pain, but it was manageable with Tylenol. After five days or so, I was on my ADD buzz. People like me must drive the drug companies nuts since they have to list all the possible side effects . . . like one may experience constipation, diarrhea, insomnia, and fatigue. It's not worth reading this stuff anymore. The energy was great in keeping the house sparkly clean for prospective buyers (yes, we are still #$@&% for sale!) and I was able to get through the workday, which was a blessing since my department was in the midst of an audit. I dropped out of yoga mostly because the sessions were too long and the twenty-minute relax-and-breathe portion agitated me. I lie there tapping fingers and feet, with racing lists in my head and probably sighing loudly instead of chanting "omm." I understand the appeal of yoga, slow, careful, methodical, but if I am going to spend an hour and a half on my body, I want to come away sweaty and feel a bit of burn in the hamstrings. Sitting on the ocean beach, listening to the surf and idle chatter with friends, an easy-read novel, and a cold drink at my side will do more on the relax meter then lying flat and still while visualizing breath coursing in and out of my body.*

We celebrated Hallie's graduation last Sunday. She graduated with honors (proud, proud) and is now getting ready to move to Chicago at the end of the summer. Robyn came home from Fredonia and left for Ireland to paint seaside landscapes for a month. The boat is in its dock space, the pool is opened, and the garden and flowers are starting to burst. It is way too busy around here to feel tired or breathe on the floor. Be well.

Hug everyone you know.
Ann

~

From: Colleen
To: Antoinette
Date: Wednesday, June 13, 2007 at 8:03 p.m.
Subject: Midway

Go Matt! We are lucky to have our steadfast men. Trade the yoga mat for a sand chair.

Colleen

~

I felt too crappy to do anything for our twenty-eighth wedding anniversary. I was too achy even for a slow boat ride. The fog and pain still lingered from the chemo and Neulasta hit. All I could do was slog through the workday, drive home, and collapse on the couch. I am getting tired of people telling me how great I am doing and how good I look when I am exhausted, weak, and cranky.

~

From: Dr. Pam
To: Antoinette
Date: Thursday, June 14, 2007 at 10:21 a.m.
Subject: Midway

So good to hear how you are fighting the fight. Good thing you have Matt as your bodyguard. I'm OK. I do have a big knot in my stomach waiting for final path results. I should find out today. I worry that they will find unclear margins and worse disease than the original biopsy. I will let you know. Please remember me to Colleen. I can't imagine how she is feeling.

Pam

~

Dr. Pam had a lumpectomy and several nodes removed. A pathology study found clear margins, no node involvement, Stage I breast cancer. All relatively good news, but her left breast also had a mass. Four sessions of an aggressive chemotherapy cocktail were prescribed. She opted for a bilateral mastectomy after treatment, after the summer. I was impressed by how quickly she pooled her professional resources and got testing, surgery, and diagnosis over and done with. Waiting was the worst part.

chapter thirty-one

Relays and Hope

The American Cancer Society Relay for Life event took place at the Sayville Middle School track field. Teams were formed, donations promised and collected, and the excitement culminated with a twenty-four-hour campout and track-walk relay. Because cancer never sleeps, each team had at least one participant on the track at all times. Besides raising money, the mission of the Relay for Life was to celebrate survivors and remember those lost. The local venue gave a face to the cancer victims. Team Colleen came out in full force.

Matt and I arrived Friday night before six o'clock. We planned not to stay long since I was flying to Chicago with Hallie in the morning. Minivans, Mercedes, and motorcycles filled the parking lots. Purple ribbons tied to the trees lining the street waved to passersby. It was a beautiful night, with clear skies promising a spectacular sunset and a cool breeze. A live band played familiar rock tunes, and tents, folding tables, and plastic chairs crowded the oval track center. Rows of porta-potties were placed on the far side. Portable night-lights stood tall on the track corner curves. Generators rumbled. Balloons tethered to tents and chairs danced in the breeze. Children dodged around the center with noisemakers. Frisbees glided through the air. White luminary paper bags lined the outside lane of the track. Each bag had a photograph and/or a name of someone who had perished from cancer on it. At dusk, the bags were lit with soft, flickering lights. I had never seen such a festive sight for such a somber cause.

We found Colleen's team in the middle of the camp. I knew she was having a very rough time. Her prognosis was not hopeful. She was terrified. Somehow, though, she had pulled together her façade and looked fabulous. Her makeup brightened her blue eyes, her nails were polished pink, and her blonde hair was styled around a tiara. She wore a pink shirt with rhinestones sparkling around the collar. Her sneakers matched the pink shade, and she made sure I noticed her glittery pink-and-white socks. I felt a little un-pinky in my pale blush polo shirt.

Team Colleen raised an incredible twenty thousand dollars!

The fashionable couple that had dropped in on the graduation party turned out to be far more interested than they initially indicated. They had returned several times to walk through the house with a designer and then an architect, ask detailed questions, and look over the pool yard. Excitement mounted when the realtor called to ask how much time we needed to move out. I said a week without thinking how that could possibly be done.

A day later, the realtor left a message letting us know that the client had made a successful bid on another house. Damn it! We realized we might need to unpack our treasures and reconsider our house-selling and home-building plans.

I was prepared to start my part-time summer school speech therapy gig in a week. The good news was that the program was less than ten miles away and ran only three hours a day for four weeks. I thought I should be able to manage fairly well. I was also excited to get back to working directly with children, even if they were not babies or toddlers.

The bad news was that our money flow during the summer would be down to a trickle. We would have to be careful, which would be difficult since there were two daughters to get back to school in September and summer was traditionally our most fun yet most costly season. We needed to sell the house!

chapter thirty-two

Chicago, Chicago

Hallie and I flew to Chicago early Saturday morning for a three-day search-for-and-secure-housing marathon. Hallie had lined up apartment and roommate interviews and signed up for an orientation at the Medill School of Journalism.

I loved Chicago. It had great culture, exciting events, and an easy-to-figure-out transportation system. Color coding worked well for me. The huge Lake Michigan could substitute as a bay even without the salty breeze and shell-beaten sands. For all that it was in the middle of the country, this city felt familiar and grounding—a suitable place for Hallie if she was going to live so far away from home.

I zigzagged the rental car through the outskirts of Chicago while Hallie navigated. Medill was in Evanston—a northern suburb of Chicago. Tree-lined streets and flowerpots blooming on the stoops added to the allure of the downtown neighborhoods. I was intrigued by the older buildings' back balconies, high ceilings, hardwood floors, and steam radiators (like the ones in my grandmother's ancient Brooklyn flat). Most of the apartments we visited had spacious rooms, modern enough kitchens, and seemingly adequate plumbing. Delightful in almost every way, except for the fact that the ones Hallie could afford were a ten- to fifteen-minute walk to any bus stop, train line, laundromat, or grocery store. I continually voiced my concern about walking home at night in the windy Chicago winter. Hallie rolled her eyes. We had more apartments to look at.

Eventually, we toured through a townhouse with four bedrooms, laundry, terrace, garage, and, a big bonus, furniture. A pool and gym facilities were included, and the bus stop and train line were less than two blocks away. Two of the young women were graduate students—one at Medill. The other roommate was the brother of one of the women, and a mechanic.

Hallie wouldn't be taking her car to Chicago—to save insurance, gas money, and probable fees for getting towed out of snow drifts. It was still a nice perk to know a handyman was nearby to fix stuff. I knew this was a sexist sentiment and wisely kept the thought to myself to avoid a debate with my daughter, who desperately wanted to make her own mark.

The girls were chatty and friendly. I got a good vibe from them, the bright rooms, and the neighborhood. The best part of the arrangement was that Renee lived only three miles away. If Hallie needed a surrogate mom or just a friendly coffee date, Renee could easily slip into that role. I could not have schemed this any better.

Hallie made the commitment. We decided to call off the other appointments and visit Renee.

Renee and Sev had a huge house on a narrow lot in a

tightly packed, tree-lined neighborhood. It was a magnificently charming home with high ceilings, meticulous woodwork, and a newly renovated kitchen. I took mental notes on the details I would like to build in my new home—if we could ever build it! I really appreciated the comfortable couch and cup of tea after a long day of traveling and apartment hunting.

Sev and Renee took us to dinner. They were enduring the angsts and fears of their oldest daughter preparing to leave for college the following month. I assured them the snarky attitudes between child and parents and the flurry of uncertainties would soon subside as they all journeyed into this new life chapter. Sev was intrigued with Hallie's search for a way to join the roller derby team in Chicago. I was hoping it was not a possibility, but Sev promised to look into it. Renee and I also listened to their political debates. Sev, a staunch conservative, and Hallie, an outspoken liberal, enjoyed a friendly exchange. Over dinner, they discussed the plight of the homeless, prison reform, and the exciting presidential primary candidates. They did not solve the nation's problems, but I was heartened that we had established a home for Hallie with wonderful people who genuinely cared for her.

The next day, Hallie and I navigated Chicago's L train. We took the Red Line from the hotel into the heart of the city and met Renee at "The Bean" in Millennium Park, strolled along the harbor, and negotiated the crowds of the Taste of Chicago fair. We got a cheap lunch out of it. We spent the rest of the day hopping on a train to get somewhere Renee thought Hallie would like and should know. What a great city. What a great day. What a great friend.

On Monday morning, Hallie insisted that I stay in the

hotel while she toured the campus and met with her department chairperson. I did not argue. Although I would have liked to see the campus, I felt sore from the walking and truly exhausted.

Halle rode the Purple Line to the Red and got off on Adams Street. She later told me that the campus was impressive, with state-of-the art equipment and technology that matched the Fox Newsroom. She also discovered that the graduate program took only seventy-two students out of hundreds of applicants. She must have done wonderful work at New Paltz to have earned herself this opportunity.

We flew back to Islip MacArthur Airport late in the afternoon—mission accomplished. I felt confident that my girl would do well in Chicago.

Robyn arrived home late Monday night. I really missed my taciturn girl. She arrived with a few bottles of Irish beer packed into her backpack alongside laundry and dried paint. She was tired, unusually chatty, and famished. I grilled her a hamburger with two slices of cheese and stayed up with her sipping a warm beer and listening to her adventures.

Overall, she'd enjoyed the trip and had a list of places to return to if she should be able to go back to Ireland. I was disappointed that she was unable to bring home her completed paintings. The program director had taken them to prepare for an art show in Cortland during the fall semester. Robyn was able to show me the pasture and cliff-side sea paintings on her camera, however. I proclaimed them to be beautiful, but she complained about her artistic skills. She was not feeling the inspiration and passion. She had reveled in the storytellers in the pubs, though.

"I thought of you, Ma. You would have loved it," she said. "A person just starts in with a story, and soon enough there's a crowd around him listening and laughing."

She was right. I would have loved that.

chapter thirty-three

Summer Days

Just when I was starting to feel like myself, treatment five closed in.

I felt fortunate that my home life swallowed a good deal of my attention and energy. Instead of being frustrated with my family and all the to-dos on my plate, I was grateful for the diversion and satisfied when I was able to cross even a few tasks off my ever-growing list. I was popping ten to twelve Tylenols a day to keep the aches in the background. I planned not to complain too much when I went in for treatment on Thursday. I was not interested in taking anything stronger than Tylenol. My adverse reactions to the few narcotics I had taken had left me foggy, careless, and depressed.

There was, however, a new and annoying symptom: hot flashes. For no apparent reason, my body temperature would rise in a wave of flush pink, starting at the top of my head and flowing down to my ankles. Lines of sweat tracked down my face, dripped from my elbows, and raced down my back and behind my knees. A wad of tissues was instantly reduced to damp pieces stuck to my cheeks and in my neck creases.

My morning coffee triggered a flash. Picking herbs from the garden and vacuuming triggered a flash. Even a cool shower after waking up in a puddle of my own juices brought on a full, drippy flash.

"Welcome to menopause," Mom quipped.

My mother had been complaining of hot flashes and night sweats for years. Years! She had gone through periods of short-tempered rants, extreme impatience, and sweat pouring down her face, followed by inconsolable chills.

One memorable, not-too-long ago episode had occurred during a Sunday dinner in the spring. Mom had insisted that the hull of my ancient Hobie Cat sailboat be removed from the side of the yard to make room for her expanding rose garden. Dad had rounded up the sons-in-law to help him lift it and move it to the opposite side of the yard. The hull had been unusable for years, but Dad insisted that there was a treasure of parts he could salvage. The sails lay buried somewhere in the garage. Mom watched and paced the back deck as the men heaved the boat from the weeds and poison ivy. Her hair blew wild in the southwesterly spring gale. Upon seeing their destination, she waved the dishtowel that was draped on her shoulder and called out, "STOP! STOP! Don't you dare crush my daffodils!"

The shrill demand of her voice barreled through the wind, stronger than any banshee could manage, frightening the men into dropping the boat. Dad, who was familiar with these outbursts, walked up to her and gently told her she was terrifying their sons-in-law. She didn't care. They were not little boys. She wanted that ugly boat out of her sight, out of her yard, far away from her daffodils. Matt later told me that he was really scared thinking that the craziness could be an inherited trait.

My summer fashion included one light layer of clothing. Stripping was not an option. I could have remained in air-conditioned rooms and surrendered my morning coffee and the occasional glass of wine at dinner to reduce the seemingly hourly flashes. But I would not sit around at home, especially during beautiful summer days. I was not about to sacrifice my only vices in this life, either. So I flashed a lot. I hoped I would be unlike my mother, and this would be a short-lived and sane symptom.

~

From: Antoinette
To: My Everyone
Date: Thursday, July 5, 2007 at 8:22 p.m.
Subject: Round Five

Round five was today. I've decided that I only like the port on chemo days. Any other time it is a nagging alien living under my skin. I don't have to love it. It will be gone as soon as these treatments are over (three more!!).

The infusion room was very busy today. There were two patients having reactions or some kind of episode that required careful attention. The nurses stayed calm and did a great job. I was so grateful my IV behaved.

On better subjects, Robyn came home from Ireland after spending a month painting Irish seascapes. She loved it. The scenery was breathtaking, the bohemian lifestyle so comfortable, and her work looks wonderful. She came home with a backpack full of laundry, a few smuggled beers, and a craving for a real hamburger. She is working at a local restaurant this summer, so we won't see much of her.

Hallie and I ventured to Chicago to apartment hunt. We drove all around Chicago and rode the train lines. It is really a great city. We found a terrific apartment in her price range, with fellow graduate students, plenty of room, natural light, and a new kitchen and washer/dryer, right on a bus line. Although this was really great, the fact that my good friend and best-ever college roommate lives less than three miles away made the choice so much greater! I feel relieved that Hallie has a local family she can call on now and then. Thanks, Renee and Sev.

Fluke fishing has been awesome in Moriches Bay. Matt has been catching regularly—delicious! Give him a call. He'll go fishing with anyone when the tides are right.

I am officially a very part-time speech therapist for the summer. I was finding the long office hours and home visits hard to juggle after the fourth chemo treatment. It's not expected to get better with the next few, so a reduced work schedule is better for everyone, including Petie, who is having difficulty waiting for anyone to come home during the sunny days. I also need more beach time. After the summer, I will be a full-time employee of Remsenburg-Speonk Elementary School. Back to speech and resource room work. I've really missed working with kids, and the school is wonderful and only a mile away from the house we cannot sell. Either we were meant to stay in Remsenburg, or we will get a buyer and I will have to close on the first day of school.

As you can see, I am trying to keep the whole cancer/chemo life on a slow back burner. It's an old Truglio trick to ignore the crisis while admiring the scenery. I am fortunate in that I will walk away from this and will soon get my body, family, friends, and life back on a "normal" path. I have truly felt all the positive energies and prayers that have been sent my way. It honestly helps. Fellow sisters, attend to your bodies, do what you have to do to make sure you remain healthy and strong. This hideous disease is more prevalent than imagined. If you are anything like me, you have no time for this nonsense. Enjoy the summer—the best season of all!

Hug everyone you know.
Antoinette

~

From: Heidi
To: Antoinette
Date: Thursday, July 5, 2007 at 9:32 p.m.
Subject: Round Five

Antoinette, thank you for keeping us updated. You are most definitely in our thoughts and prayers. Chin up. You are doing great!

Heidi

~

From: Sherry
To: Antoinette
Date: Thursday, July 5, 2007 at 10:12 p.m.
Subject: Round Five

I was just thinking of you! Thanks for adding me to your e-mail list. When I was having a hard time, Janet kept telling me, "This will end. This will end." Keep it in mind even when it feels like forever.

Sherry

From: Julie
To: Antoinette
Date: Thursday, July 5, 2007 at 10:23 p.m.
Subject: Round Five

Hey, girlfriend, I love your email updates—very inspirational. You are a wonderful writer. Will we see you this weekend at Davis Park? Dave got his Sunfish on the beach and wants to practice this weekend. He is psyched for the Labor Day race and is determined to beat ANYONE with the last name Martin! Love you,

Julie

From: Antoinette
To: Julie
Date: Friday, July 6, 2007 at 1:41 p.m.
Subject: Round Five

Tell Dave to "bring it!" I may be dealing with this poisoning, but I'll be damned if a Sunfish with a prettier sail than mine beats me! We will be there on Saturday for the day. See you then. Love, hugs, and kisses.

Ann

The Fourth of July landed on a Wednesday, which postponed our usual holiday beach festivities to the weekend. I looked forward to seeing Dr. Pam. She and her family were traveling from their home in Pennsylvania to spend an extended weekend at their Davis Park beach house. She had an oceanfront beach house that had been in her family close to fifty years. So many of the cottagey homes in the community were built by families looking for a "far away getaway so close to home."

The original beach houses were rugged, with minimal accommodations. Water was pumped from a well, and gas lights and gas refrigerators were standard. Bathing suits and T-shirts were washed in a tub and hung on clothesline to dry in the sunny, salty breeze. It was far from a resort vacation, barely a step up from camping in a tent or boat. But Dr. Pam and Pam B. would not have traded their childhood summers for anything else. They were free to run through the reeds, swim in the ocean, sail on the bay, beachcomb for shells and hazy beach glass, dig clams, and pull blue claw crabs from a string with a raw chicken wing for bait from the harbor docks.

Over the years, the community was developed. More modern houses were built. Electric and water services were made available. A volunteer fire department, U.S. Post Office (opened Monday through Friday from July 1 to Labor Day, 11:00 a.m. to 2:00 p.m.), Suffolk County police station, convenient harbor store, hopping restaurant and bar, and Catholic church—complete with confession and Mass schedules—made the community into a full-fledged summer town.

Fire Island has several summer communities that are accessible only by sea, with more shops, bars, stylish homes, and reliable ferry services, but simple Davis Park was our favorite. Our old friends who shared our beach and bay passions were there. Our kids loved it.

During this shortened holiday weekend, Sara, Hallie, and Robyn had work and had made plans with their friends, so I packed a cooler and one beach bag for a day trip to Davis Park. Matt and I took our motorboat. We planned to stay for the day and leave before sunset, missing the costume party. Little compromises had to be endured.

We left early and rode through the calm, meandering channel of Moriches Bay. An occasional small boat drifted into the waterway as we slowly cruised along, and we waved to the fisherman.

"Fluke fishing has been great," Matt called over the loud rumble of the outboard engine.

"Maybe tomorrow," I offered as a consolation. I wanted to get to Davis Park. I hoped to be able to pull my Sunfish from the beach and sail before I parked myself in a sand chair with my friends—and before the wind blew too hard. I was not sure if I could manage my little boat in a strong wind. My Sunfish resided at the beach in front of the Bensons', and they let me keep the sails, daggerboard, and rudder on the side of their house.

I loved my Sunfish. I'd had one since I was twelve years old. The beauty of this fourteen-foot monohull boat was that I could easily rig and handle it by myself. When I was a kid, Dad bought a used Sunfish and built a lift with a hand crank. During my teen summers, my three sisters and one friend would pile onto the little boat and I would sail it the five miles across the bay to Barrett Beach or Sailors Haven, saving us the dollar ferry fare. We stuffed our towels into a plastic garbage bag. Diana, my middle sister, diligently bailed the small cockpit with a cut-out Clorox bottle. Little Barbara hung onto the bow chock cleat, whooping as waves crashed over her and into her mouth. She dared not let go, since I warned her I was not good at man-overboard maneuvers and we didn't have life jackets.

I often wondered why my mother allowed us to do this on a regular basis. She must have known of the dangers, since she would never allow my baby brother, Billy, to join us. My sister Mary and I each had only one season of lessons at the local Wet Pants Sailing Club under our belts. Mary quickly became bored with the whims of the fickle winds and jumped at the chance to operate motorboats. But sailing was my definition of freedom.

I was never very skilled in understanding and applying terms and had no heart for the competitive demands of racing. Instead, I preferred to sail by feel and practice. I loved the quiet with just the wind and the lapping of the waves against the sides of the hull. I loved the challenge of not getting to a destination in a straight line, tweaking the mainsheet, leaning my body out on the windward side with my feet holding under the hiking strap to balance the hull on its side as I quickly skimmed up and down turbulent waves. When I could shake my sisters loose, I took my Sunfish out just to sail around, rehearse my awful poetry out loud, and sing. While Matt and I were dating, I frequently sailed out to his clamming spot on the porgy bar to bring him brownies and steal a few private minutes with him on the deck of his small clam boat before heading back to the mainland in time to report to work.

My Sunfish was now fourteen years old. Despite its age, the hull was dry and light. I'd taught my girls, as well as a few of their beach friends, how to sail on it, and had once organized a junior class for the Labor Day Davis Park Regatta. I'd splurged on a plain white racing sail several years before so that I could head the boat upwind as close as possible. Fun memories.

A light wind from the southwest blew along the cove where we moored the boat. It would be a perfect day for a sail. I saw Dr. Pam waving at us from the Bensons' deck as Matt set the anchor. She was always up early. Sailing would have to wait for another perfect day.

Dr. Pam and I hugged and cried on the deck.

"You look good, Ann," she said. "I really mean it. I am not just saying it."

"And you look terrific," I replied with conviction.

She pulled one of my short curls. "You are so lucky to have so much hair."

I stroked both of my hands over her baby-fine strawberry blonde bob. "You will get through this and be able to walk away with brand-new hair and perky boobs."

Matt and I spent most of the day sitting in low sand chairs under a cheery umbrella on the ocean side. We stretched our legs and dug our feet into the warm sand while the constant rush and fall of the surf lulled us into a peaceful state. Matt soon leaned his chair back and finally relaxed. Dr. Pam staked her family next to us with bright umbrellas, well-seasoned beach chairs, and a giant basket filled with sand toys and paddle games. We nibbled on pretzel rods and sipped beer in cozies.

Young Lisa, tall and graceful even with her little boy clutching her leg, joined us. A white do-rag was wrapped around her head. I was startled by how plain she looked without eyelashes and eyebrows or a hint of a hairline around her ears. Her port appeared to stick out more angrily than mine.

Colleen and her husband, Eric, walked the beach from their rental on the east side of the community and joined our circle. Colleen had been in extreme pain and felt very slow. A rainbow of drugs kept her functional, but she claimed that being on the beach was the best medicine.

The wind picked up. The sky reflected a hazy blue on the ocean that roared as it rolled toward us. Dr. Pam's children challenged the surf with boogie boards while Lisa's little one held his daddy's hand and jumped the trailing wash on the shore.

We commiserated about our journeys thus far and the expected outcomes. Dr. Pam would begin a regime of four aggressive chemotherapy treatments and return to surgery for a double mastectomy and reconstruction in the fall. Lisa had already had a unilateral mastectomy and had just finished her chemotherapy protocol. She still, however, had months of treatment ahead. She'd purposely skipped her fortieth birthday in April.

"I'm having a birthday bash in October—the half-year mark," she said. "You all have to come!"

Colleen had to take a leave of absence from her position in the county parks department. We were all saddened to hear that when she saw her doctor's prognosis on the disability paperwork, it read *terminal.* Terminal! What a horrid word to spell out on paper. Mustering hope and strength with that on her medical and work records took unbelievable resolve and courage.

We recounted our fears of the unknown, our rage, our worries about our kids, husbands, and parents with tears, laughs, and hands clasped together. The ocean continued to crash forward, drowning our words, taking our fears out to sea to mix with the ocean's life forces, leaving us with ourselves—raw and determined to battle on for the sake of our own selves, our tomorrows with those we love, and the lives in which we still had so much to do. The tide crept closer to our chairs. It was time for a swim in the wild sea, to jump between and under the crests, float on calmed waves, and then return to shore, refreshed and renewed.

chapter thirty-four

Plowing Forward

From: Colleen
To: Antoinette
Date: Wednesday, July 18, 2007 at 9:17 a.m.
Subject: Play Date

How are you feeling? I propose a play date. I'm putting together an "invite only" karaoke night at the Sayville Inn this Friday . . . it's going to be a lot of laughs . . . which is just what we cancer ladies need. Want to come? Pammie is coming. 8:00 in the back building, $25 per person to cover the room and, sorry, cash bar. Hope you can make it!

From: Antoinette
To: Colleen
Date: Wednesday, July 18, 2007 at 11:22 a.m.
Subject: Play Date

I have to see where I am on Friday. My friend is taking me to a Reiki session with her in the afternoon.I think it is yoga-ish (even though I like the theoryand can read up on these spiritual practices, I can't seem to embrace them).I agreed to go when she promised that no one will touch me. She also promised gyros afterward. I have to make a huge pot of chowder on Friday night. Brooklyn and parts of New Jersey will be depleted of most of their Italians since they will be at my parents' house for the annual family picnic on Saturday. I will try to make it to karaoke, but no promises. Is it ladies only? You know that Nick only sings when he has a few or a lot, and Matt should never sing no matter what his blood alcohol level is.

Ann

~

From: Colleen
To: Antoinette
Date: Wednesday, July 18, 2007 at 4:42 p.m.
Subject: Play Date

Let me know how you make out with Reiki. I'd do just about anything for a gyro. Leave Friday night open-ended. Eric and some of our other guys will be there. Right now, I'm going where the laughter is; some people follow the light, I follow the chuckles. Keep in touch and be strong, my friend. The end of chemo is on the horizon. XXOO

Colleen

I tired too easily. The summer school had so many stairs to climb as I picked up and returned children from their speech therapy sessions. My knees and back screamed when I finally reached home and fell into the ancient Adirondack chair on the patio. Petie was disappointed with our short walks, but between his coughing and my fatigue, a stroll up to the corner and back was enough for both of us. I did not make it to karaoke.

My friend Anne St. John had taken me to a Reiki session. Anne had been having a very rough time dealing with a messy divorce after a twenty-five-year marriage. Always steady and practical, the anxiety and anger overwhelmed her. She began practicing yoga to relieve the crippling tension and was the one who had encouraged me to really try it as well. Disappointed that I did not find relief, Anne recommended Reiki, claiming it was wonderful.

Reiki is an ancient therapeutic technique that uses hovering hands to heal and provide comfort. I was more open to it when Anne explained that the therapist did not touch the body.

We went together. I lay on a table surrounded by dim light and soothing, yogi-type music—I asked for the incense to be removed—while the very nice therapist quietly drifted her hands over me. It was interesting, different, a little weird—okay, very weird. I did, however, enjoy the lunch Anne and I shared afterward at the Turkish restaurant nearby. It was always fun to catch up with her.

The next day was the family picnic. Each summer, one Saturday was devoted to the event, which my parents host in their vast yard on the Great South Bay. Crowds of aunts, uncles, grandparents, cousins, and old friends who might as well be family traveled from nearby neighborhoods, Brooklyn, New Jersey, Maryland, and sometimes California and

Oregon. They converged on Palmer Drive, parking on the front lawn and along the curvy street or, weather permitting, arriving by boat, for a day of jumping from the dock into the bay, water skiing (if the bay was calm enough and if there was a fast enough boat), grilling, and playing games of bocce in the backyard and volleyball in the front yard using the parked cars as boundaries. We ate continuously. The big yard had shade for the circles of grandmas and grand-aunties who sat on lawn chairs and gently rocked strollers to coax babies to nap.

Most of the hundred or so family members were related to my father's side. Two to three generations of Italians could trace their American beginnings within a few-mile radius in Brooklyn. My parents were some of the first of their generation to emigrate to the suburbs on Long Island or New Jersey. Their house was perfect for the volume and activities.

There was always too much food set out on the patio tables and cluttering the kitchen counters. Homemade and bakery-bought sweets covered the dining room table. Everyone had a specialty to bring. Uncle Phil brought bread and rolls from Brooklyn, Aunt Linda cooked four trays of her sausage and peppers, Mom made her meatballs and ziti, Aunt Betty brought fried chicken—the list was endless.

Since my grandmother's passing, I had been cooking her Manhattan clam chowder. Grandma had instructed me on the ingredients, the sequencing, and the seasoning. Actually, I asked questions, and she let me watch how she made it. Grandma was an amazing cook. She could transform freezer-burnt broccoli into a gourmet masterpiece. She never wrote down or measured anything, but she always invited anyone interested to watch and learn. Over the years, my chowder slowly evolved as my own. I used my freshly made pesto, fennel instead of celery, crushed tomatoes instead of tomato juice, and the water from the clams instead of bottled clam juice. But no matter how I changed the recipe, it was always called Grandma's Clam Chowder—a treasured compliment. For this year's Family Picnic Day, I cooked up a fragrant batch in my largest pot.

For almost forty years the sun had almost always shined down on Family Picnic Day. This day gave us all a chance to see each other, catch up, reminisce, celebrate the milestones, and remember those who had passed on. This year we counted eighty-seven people in the yard. My girls, nieces and nephews, and cousins and their families all joined us. It wasn't too hard to keep a smile pasted on my face all day, even when I had to repeat the highlights of my treatments and explain the obvious port to each of my aunts.

Grandma used to say that our family was so rich in flesh. We had so many in our lives we had loved and who had known us from the beginning. She felt sorry for those families poor in flesh with no history and too few relations in their lives and hearts.

From: Antoinette
To: Dr. Pam
Date: Wednesday, July 25, 2007 at 8:49 p.m.
Subject: Good Luck!

Thinking of you. Drink lots of water, add a teaspoon of Metamucil, and have Jolly Rancher Sours on hand and your good man by your side. It should all be smooth going. I went today, took a nap, and now I'm up. No drama this time. I resolved to ignore the port discomfort. I can call next month to get it removed after the last treatment! Vacation starts soon; I can taste it! When will you guys be there?

Be strong, Pam. Today, it may feel bleak and sad and way too scary, but in no time it is over and you walk away from it. Let me know how you are doing.

Hug everyone you know.
Ann

From: Antoinette
To: My Everyone
Date: Thursday, July 26, 2007 at 6:22 p.m.
Subject: Round Six

Six chemo sessions are done!If my math is correct, only two more to go. No drama this time. I didn't pass out on the nurse when she poked the port. It felt so real that the end is near when I scheduled the last session for Aug 31 without the follow-up Neulasta shot. I should be in sailing form for the Davis Park Regatta on Labor Day. I tried a Reiki session (healing touch) with my friend Anne. It was different. Thanks,

Hug Everyone You Know

Anne, it is always fun to spend time and new experiences with you.

In the meantime, we signed up with a new real estate group. We are renting storage space to put the stuff that has been packed in boxes for eighteen months. This weekend's chore was to get most of the garage and basement cleared. Closets are another matter.

We had our family picnic last week. A troop of aunts, uncles, cousins, and old friends came to my parents' house with too much food (we are of the belief that if there is not enough left over to feed everyone for three more days, then someone surely went home hungry). I think relatives and friends who had not seen me since treatments were relieved to see me looking well (hair and a light tan) with an up attitude. We caught up on family gossip, marveled at how much the babies have grown, congratulated engagements, patted my cousin's latest baby under construction, played in the bay—a very fun day. The north wind offered water-ski opportunities, except for me. I'll be ready next year!

We are looking forward to our beach week at Davis Park. No better respite than to be in the sight and earshot of the ocean, a simple cottage to call home for a week, no driving, great friends, and the biggest worry being if we have enough rum and gin.
Enjoy this wonderful summer.

Hug everyone you know.
Antoinette

From: Chris Flaherty
To: Antoinette
Date: Thursday, July 26, 2007 at 7:56 p.m.
Subject: Round Six

So glad you are feeling good. I cannot wait until we are together at the beach! I am so ready for a vacation. Sean reminded me of how he cannot wait until you feed him and David at the beach. They love your eggplant! We'll make sure they don't tire you out. Talk to you soon!

Chris

From: Dr. Pam
To: Antoinette
Date: Thursday, July 26, 2007 at 8:09 p.m.
Subject: Good Luck!

Well, I finished my chemo just fine. Got lots of premeds and it went smoothly. Felt a little carsick last night, not much appetite, but ate like a horse tonight. I just tossed back a beer. I got my Neulasta shot today. I can't wait for the beach. Hugs to all.

Pam

From: Sara
To: Mom
Date: Thursday, July 26, 2007 at 11:48 p.m.
Subject: Round Six

Love you, Mom. See you soon.

chapter thirty-five

Beach Week

The cozy two-bedroom cottage sat in the middle of Pepperidge Walk, just up the boardwalk from the Flahertys' and Kovaricks' rentals and the Bensons' bayfront house. The Kureys were one walk over, and the Hofmiesters were settled in their rental on the eastern end of the community. For almost twenty years, we had all taken our summer vacations during the first week of August.

While Matt and I arrived by boat, laden with coolers, boxes of groceries and liquor, boogie boards, surfboards, fishing gear, umbrellas, and sand chairs, the Flahertys and Kovaricks piled their kids and a mound of boxes and containers onto the ferry. It took an amazing feat of physics and bungee cords to pack their stuff into several carts and pull them the quarter of a mile along the boardwalk to Pepperidge Walk.

I looked forward to an extra fun and relaxing week. I prepared and organized, precooked and froze batches of tomato sauce, pulled pork, and chicken cutlets for easy meal preparations. I also brought along the fixings for my eggplant stacks, which David Kurey and Sean Flaherty had been asking for since school let out.

We spent the first Beach Week afternoon unpacking and helping the Flahertys and Kovaricks manage their wares into their nearby rentals. I may like to cook special meals on vacation, but the Kovaricks had stepped up their game and brought their recipe files for the week, along with detailed seasonings, specialized gadgets, and their own smoked fish and infused oils. Dan collected his homegrown peppers of varying heat, and Coll asked Matt if the crab traps were set. She wanted to try a new recipe: citrus crab quesadillas. Nothing was set yet, so David and Sean retrieved the trap, took a chicken leg and two wings from someone's freezer, and paddled a kayak to the spot Matt directed.

This was the perfect place to truly relax. The cottage we had rented was cheerful, with natural light streaming in from all directions, comfortable furniture, shady front and back decks, and a simple working kitchen. The music of the ocean played in the background. The sand held shell and beach glass treasures to collect during our beach walks. I took guiltless afternoon naps under the shade of an umbrella or cooling fan in the bedroom. The salt air and sea sounds could lull me into a deep sleep for over an hour—such a needed decadence.

We spent our days and nights on the beaches, sharing meals, telling old stories, and keeping tabs on the kids as they freely moved from house to house playing games and finding innocent mischief. At sunset, we met on the Bensons' deck. Champagne flutes were filled. We all watched as the sun dipped into the western horizon through billowy clouds, sending golden pink rays across the sky and onto a still bay.

We lifted our glasses—a salute to an exhausting, fun-filled day with loving friends. "It's good to be us," we toasted.

I felt so well.

Dr. Pam had started chemotherapy a few days before vacation. Tufts of her fine hair blew away in the wind. She asked our beach neighbor, a professional photographer, to take her family's annual Christmas portrait before she lost more. The handsome family posed on the bayside wearing white shirts and wide, bright smiles that accented their pink tans. Even the dog smiled.

Matt, Dr. Pam, and I went to visit Terry. She was out of the hospital, happily recovering at her beloved beach house. Tall and stately, Terry claimed to be doing well even though she had to limit her time in the sun. I was taken aback by the absence of her brown ponytail, which until recently had reached midway down her back, and her winter-white complexion. Despite the grueling treatments she'd been undergoing, however, she'd been walking every day and keeping up with the Davis Park community politics and her growing brood of grandchildren. The treatments were working, and she felt hopeful.

Dr. Pam and I quickly recapped our cancer episodes. Terry showed Dr. Pam how to effortlessly tie a do-rag on her head. She and Matt shared fishing reports. It felt eerily normal, despite the cancer in the room.

We had a real offer. Not the price we'd hoped for, but Matt crunched the numbers, and it was good enough.

Before returning the realtor's call, Matt looked straight at me and asked, "Are you sure you want to do this? You will have a twenty-five-minute commute to work from Sayville, the fishing is not as good in the Great South Bay, and building a house is stressful."

Was he kidding? My commute would be in the opposite direction of traffic—a decompression commute. Besides, living in the same community where I taught could be tricky when it came to budget debates, board member campaigns, and students recognizing me in the grocery store aisles and exiting the liquor store. Selling the house and building a new home in Sayville would enable us to be mortgage and loan free—now *that* was freedom! We would be closer to our families and the dear friends we loved to play with. We could build the home we had been planning for almost two years. A home with high ceilings and a kitchen we could both fit in and work in together; long, sunny windows that would let in natural light; an efficient heating system; a master bedroom on the ground floor so we could grow old without having to negotiate steps with aging knees and backs; a tidy yard that would not sap all energies and time; and no pool to upkeep. If Matt had to fish in Moriches Bay, then we could afford a dock space there.

Stress? I knew stress. Showing and selling a house for two years was stressful. Raising three girls into adulthood was very stressful. Our families produced streams of stress, and our jobs featured an endless parade of stress. Cancer was stressful. But I preferred to think of life's stressors as a series of adventures. One slogs through stress, but adventure can be enlightening, exciting, a real trip. An adventure, even a rotten one, has its highlights and beauty. Sometimes, an epiphany can emerge and life becomes richer and more amazing.

"Let's go on this adventure. Let's build a home. Let's say *yes*!"

Contracts would be ready in a week.

❋

chapter thirty-six

Sick and Tired of This Crap

I was back in the infusion chair a week after I left the beach. Matt picked me up in the mid-afternoon for the seventh chemo hit. I was anxious about this appointment since I had gotten a call from Memorial Sloan Kettering a few days before explaining that Dr. Sheren had to take personal time. Could I see her associate—who, they assured me, was hailed as an excellent doctor—or would I rather postpone treatment for a week?

Although I was not comfortable having someone new probing me, I assumed that my regular nurse, Rose Ann, who was sympathetic toward my squeamish ways, would be present. I could deal with that. I did not want to manage the other arrangements rescheduling a treatment would require.

When the day came, Rose Ann was not available. Matt reminded the new nurse I needed the "brown needle" for the port.

That's my good man, I thought, *always paying attention.*

Both the substitute doctor and nurse were very nice and very chatty. This must be a good technique to reassure and calm a patient; it probably works well for most people. But I was not up for conversation. I dutifully answered the direct questions—"How is the fatigue?" "How is the pain?"—but when he asked an open-ended question ("How are you doing through all this?"), all I could answer was, "Fine, I'm fine, really."

I hoped the very nice doctor would take the hint, but he had wisdom and experience to share. I tried to be polite and not close my eyes while he talked. The nurse narrated the port stabbing, drew blood, and taped the tube in place. As the doctor continued talking, typing his notes with one finger, Matt saw I was about to pass out. He caught me before the table slipped out from under me. While they laid me flat on the table, Matt calmly explained that this was normal. "She really is fine."

The nurse retook my vitals. I sipped cold water. The doctor asked, "Are you up for the chemo today?"

Matt and I simultaneously chimed, "Yes!"

The doctor had a few more wise tidbits to share while waiting for my color to come back. The blood count report came back with normal levels. We were good to go.

The infusion room hummed with quiet activity. I settled into a lounge chair while a nurse plugged me into the poison and offered me a warm blanket. Matt rummaged through my tote bag and pulled out a house design magazine with orange Post-it tabs poking out along the edges. He handed me my iPod and goofy sleeping mask.

I noticed a familiar woman settling into a station across from me. She was a short, round woman with a well-fitted brunette wig in a bobbed style.

Over the past few months, I had become astute in identifying a head wearing a wig. Like a terrible toupee, a bad wig sat stiff, and usually had an outrageous style and color. A good wig's color and cut complimented the face rather than giving the wearer an excuse to experiment with punky headdresses and colors not found in nature. If I had to go with a wig, I thought I would choose one that was close to my usual color and style rather than shock myself and everyone else with a whole new look while going through treatment.

I had seen this woman in the infusion room a few times. She appeared to be about my age and was very fashionable. The hairs on her wig flowed with her head movements and seemed to comfortably fit her expressions and actions. Her makeup was always well blended, with careful attention paid to the eye shadow shades that complemented her light brown eyes and Ann Taylor ensembles. Her lipstick, fingernails, and even toenails, peeking out of kitten-heeled sandals, all matched.

Each time I saw this woman, she was accompanied by a man of the same age dressed in a sharp business suit, a sister or perhaps a friend also dressed in office attire, and a young woman, who looked about my Robyn's age, in a camp counselor uniform. The woman would mold herself into a recliner and sweetly recite her full name and birthdate to the nurse. Once she was plugged in, one of her people would tuck a warm blanket around her while the others positioned chairs around her, holding her hand, rubbing her shoulders, and whispering niceties.

This time, the entourage included another young adult (maybe Sara's age) and two other fiftyish women, all of whom were dressed for a day in a professional office. There were too many people to huddle in the small station, but the back of the infusion room had a larger space that offered privacy. A nurse wheeled the woman, reclined and warmly tucked into the chair, to the back area. The man followed close behind, pushing the IV pole, while the others joined the parade with chairs in hand. Someone took the cookie basket off the shelf.

I could not and would not speculate on the pain and terror this family must be going through. I knew firsthand that looking great was deceptive during the physical and emotional punishment of illness and treatment. If physical closeness and encouraging affirmations from loved ones who'd taken time from their day to be there offered this woman comfort while she was taking a chemo hit, then so be it.

This was not my way of coping, however. The less attention and verbiage I gave this cancer, the less real it was in my day. This cancer was nothing more than a detour—not a chronic condition or terminal illness. Audible words, long dialogues, and ownership would provide it with an embodiment. I tried to keep that to a minimum. The treatment I was willingly putting myself through was aimed to kill any trace of cancer that might have been left behind from surgery. I believed it was completely gone, and the chemo and radiation therapies served as insurance against a recurrence. This cancer did not deserve an audience and would never be referred to with the personal pronoun *my.*

Matt sat looking through the magazine and nibbling on a cookie. He was all the audience I needed. His role was security. He made sure I was comfortable and that no one made me cry. He stood by as a quiet observer—large, stoic, ready to pounce. My job was to soldier through as bravely as my wimpy self could do and always look forward.

Matt jotted notes on Post-its. I shut down my iPod and pulled my goofy mask over my eyes. The damn port throbbed.

~

From: Antoinette
To: My Everyone
Date: Thursday, August 16, 2007 at 7:35 p.m.
Subject: One More to Go

Greetings, wonderful friends and family! After today's treatment, I am down to just one more. Today, I had a substitute doctor and nurse since my regular team had a personal day. I was not willing to reschedule since it would only cause a domino effect with the rest of my scheduled appointments and life events. With the heightened anxiety due to this temporary change, Matt caught me before I passed out onto the floor and explained that this was normal. I recovered quickly, albeit embarrassed. Good white blood count. The actual infusion was uneventful, and I was out of the chair by 3:30. We stopped for crab cakes on the way home, and then I took a nap. DONE!

The last Neulasta shot is tomorrow. My last treatment was scheduled so I would not miss any work in my new position at Remsenburg-Speonk. It is the day before the Davis Park Regatta. Since I will not need a Neulasta shot, I should be in decent sailing and costume kayak "race" shape. My circle of beach pals has been hit hard with the breast cancer beast. Four of us have been battling this year. We are planning a "brilliant" kayak float complete with pink boas, pinker hats, and "Fight Like a Girl" logos.

We had a wonderful beach vacation last week with our regular beach pals. Lots of sun, the ocean was just beautiful, some sailing (the wind was "wicked" and my little Sunfish was frequently airborne), fishing, loads of freshly dug clams, summer reading, and fireworks!

The big news is WE SOLD THE HOUSE!!! It had to happen. We planted our best garden ever, a statue of St. Joseph was buried upside down among the basil and sunflowers, and I got the final confirmation for the Remsenburg-Speonk position. We have a contract signed and sealed. We had to drop the price substantially, but our buyer is paying cash, in dollars. It's enough. Since the buyer will be overseas for a few months, we are not closing until November—plenty of time to pack up Hallie and Robyn for school and pack and throw away so much crap. I can't wait to order the hugest dumpster possible. Matt and I will be moving in with my parents while we secure the permits and build our new home in Sayville. 2008 is destined to be an exciting adventure.

I am keeping the laughs above the anxiety while looking forward and appreciating the scenery along the way. I'm fine . . . really.

Hug everyone you know.
Antoinette

From: Dr. Pam
To: Antoinette
Date: Friday, August 17, 2007 at 6:51 a.m.
Subject: One More to Go

Loved your note. I go today for Chemo #2. I am OK with all the poking and prodding, but, remember, I'm a doctor—it's what I do. I hope my counts are OK. I feel pretty good, just a little cough. I got my head shaved on Monday. It feels better and I am not so messy. Well, off to eat my breakfast and my premeds.

Pam

~

From: Addie
To: Antoinette
Date: Friday, August 17, 2007 at 9:18 a.m.
Subject: One More to Go

Bravo! Keep these notes. Your attitude will someday help millions! Thinking of you in love and prayer.

Addie

~

From: Gingerbread House; Joi Nobisso
To: Antoinette
Date: Friday, August 17, 2007 at 11:34 a.m.
Subject: One More to Go

Oh, my gracious! You have the most positive and wonderful and loving spirit! So many people would buckle under rather than fight against this beast, but you conquer it with love and good humor! If you're ever choosing teams, I'll be waving at you like mad, "Pick me! Pick me!"

I went to a yard sale recently and asked for children's books. The lady tells me, "Oh, I save all of those! I'm a teacher." When I told her I write kids' books, she suddenly "remembers" that I went to her school, and she starts squealing and hugging and kissing me. All the while, I'm thinking, "Wow. My mind really IS going! Who is this?" Then she says, "The kids loved your Famous Seaweed Soup!" AH! That explains why she loved me so much: I was you.

I am keeping you in my heart and prayers! BIG, BIG hugs, and lots of love,

Joi

From: Antoinette
To: Joi Nobisso
Date: Friday, August 17, 2007 at 4:53 p.m.
Subject: One More to Go

Thanks for the encouraging words, Joi. I am so honored to be mistaken as you.

chapter thirty-seven

Adventurous Stress

My patience was wearing thin. It might have been the chemo talking, but I couldn't wait for the girls to leave for school. All I wanted them to do was pack and label boxes for the storage garage. Their bedroom floors and the downstairs rooms were littered with books, forgotten dolls, dusty trophies, and piles of seemingly useless papers. I told them if they did not take care of it, their unclaimed, unboxed, unlabeled things would be at my mercy; I had a twenty-yard dumpster in the driveway and was not afraid to use it! But they all seemed intent on ignoring me, and making my life more difficult while they were at it.

It all started with Hallie. She insisted on driving to New Paltz for a weekend to visit friends she would not see for a long time. She drove off on a hot Friday afternoon in her little Dodge Spirit. Matt's suggestion to check tire pressure, oil, and water levels were ignored. Matt had taught the girls the basics of car maintenance. Sara and Robyn had embraced the skill. They didn't mind crouching down to monitor tire pressure or pulling out a dipstick to check the oil, but Hallie preferred not to get her hands dirty and relied on eyeing the tire inflation and dashboard warning lights.

Hallie called while I was taping and labeling boxes in the garage.

"Mommy! Mommy!" she sobbed over the phone.

My heart sank, and a sickening wave of nausea washed through me. "What happened? Are you hurt? Where are you?"

"Daddy's yelling at me," she cried.

"What? Why?"

"My car is on fire, and he is yelling at me!"

Less than ten minutes before, Hallie had called Matt at his office to ask if she should be worried about the smoke coming out of the hood.

"The engine light is on," she reported while driving sixty-five miles an hour on the New York Thruway.

"Pull over! Pull over!" Matt shouted.

"I think I can make it to the service station," she said.

Matt hollered louder. "No! Just pull over NOW!"

Hallie hung up, leaving Matt desperately dialing and re-dialing her number. When she finally picked up the phone again, she said, "Dad, I pulled over, and now there are flames coming out of the hood. What should I do?"

"Get out of the fucking car! Now! Get OUT!" He was hoarse with panic.

"But what about my equipment, the EZ Pass?" she asked. Before he could repeat his directives, she announced that a state trooper and fire truck had pulled up in front of her. She hung up again.

"Wait, Hallie, let me talk to someone," Matt shouted from one hundred miles away.

The little Dodge Spirit was destroyed. The engine and dashboard melted into a molten mess. Smoldering plumes of gray clouds created a fog on the Thruway. Burnt rubber and oil wafted through the sticky summer afternoon. Two fire trucks and several state troopers were hailed. A news helicopter reported a five-mile backup on the northbound Thruway just above the Tappan Zee Bridge.

Hallie answered questions and provided her license. A trooper retrieved insurance and registration cards and the EZ Pass from the glove compartment. Because Hallie had such a sweet smile, he also saved her roller derby equipment bag from the backseat. A friend picked her up, and her boyfriend offered to get her from New Paltz, since Matt and I separately told her to take a train home.

That, too, proved to be a debacle. The boyfriend, though attentive and accommodating, ran out of gas between Thruway service stations. I checked the calendar: fifteen more days until I would put her on the plane to Chicago.

The following Friday, Robyn picked up her freshly tuned bicycle in Bellport—and drove my Caravan into a curb, banging up the tire rim and brakes system, which turned out to be a very expensive problem, not to mention an ill-timed one. We were to drive her to Buffalo the next day. I thought of renting a van, but my sister Mary saved the day and offered her minivan for the weekend.

I was not feeling confident about Robyn's transfer to the University of Buffalo. It was a huge campus; it would be so easy for her to feel lost and alone. She had been more elusive than usual the whole summer. She'd come to the beach and to family functions, but reluctantly. When we announced the good news about the house sale, she shrugged and claimed that she would not miss the house or the neighborhood. She packed one large Rubbermaid container to take to my parents' basement and fit her college life in one other.

"That's it?" I asked.

"I don't need much, Ma," she replied, hooking her bike rack to Mary's minivan hatch. It had taken all summer to drag her to the outlets to buy jeans and boots. I stuffed newly bought packs of underwear and wool socks into her Buffalo-bound container.

We left for Buffalo at five in the morning. The ten-hour journey droned long and tiresome. Robyn barely spoke. She worried me. It was difficult to really talk with her, so I wrote her a letter and planned to leave it in plain sight before we left her.

~

Sweetheart,

You are about to embark on the second year of your college career. It's a career because at this point in your life, getting a degree is your primary job. You have three short years to develop skills that qualify you to do something other than wait on tables. In today's world, a woman is at a significant disadvantage without an education she can apply to the real world. I admire the courage in you I never had. But you need a plan. Experiencing the world with even a small plan enriches the adventure and your life.

I am not too worried about your general well-being. Last year, you proved that you can take care of yourself and showed responsibility in completing your classwork. I am, however, concerned that you do not move beyond the requirements. Passion takes work, no matter how much innate talent you have, no matter how much you love it. You have to own it. This year I charge you to find that passion, declare a course of study that would reflect that passion, give it purpose, dive in, play in it, and love it. Three years of study is a very short time.

I love you, baby. Words pale at the depth of this mommy-love. Do great this year. Brush your teeth and your hair, every day. Be well (eat at least one fruit a day and poop once a day). Be happy (only you have the power to make you happy) and be good! Love you fiercely with all my heart and soul.

Mommy

Typical of western New York weather, Buffalo welcomed and bid us farewell with pouring rain complete with thunder and lightning.

While we were still driving home, Robyn left a message on the home answering machine.

"Okay, Mom," she said. "Love you, too."

The naps I was taking, though necessary, were getting in my way. Between packing up the house, getting Robyn and Hallie off to school, and preparing for the new job and Labor Day weekend, I was getting frustrated with the chemo fatigue and aches. I had to keep reminding myself that there was just one more chemo session to go and I did not have room for a postponement if my counts were low. Even though I was cranky about it, each day I took an hour-and-a-half nap with Petie cuddled next to me, and I surrendered the day by nine o'clock. Frustrating.

I had met the radiologist at Sloan Kettering back in March. Both Matt and I were very pleased with the attention she gave my questions and concerns. She recommended starting the sessions one month after the completion of chemotherapy. That seemed fair. She explained the science behind the treatment (not that I really understood it, but I appreciated the patience) and the daily protocol. It would take five to six weeks. I should expect fatigue and skin burns, but she assured me that being a rather strong and healthy woman, I should fare well.

As September drew near, Matt and I realized that the forty-five-minute drive to Commack and probable hour or more back to Remsenburg in the midst of rush-hour traffic on the Long Island Expressway would just compound the side effects of radiation. I planned to go by myself since the daily zapping took all of five minutes. Matt did not need to adjust his schedule just to sit in a waiting room. My radiologist and oncologist agreed that receiving the radiation therapy at a facility closer to work and home made sense. I made a few calls and settled on a radiology facility fifteen minutes from my new job and our current home.

Our buyer negotiated the closing for early November. This extra time gave me the opportunity to settle into my new position and get through most of the radiation therapy. It also gave us plenty of time to clear the house out and clean up the yard. We would be able to harvest our abundant tomato crop before the closing date, and I should be done with radiation by then, too.

We were packing in higher gear now that we had a timeline. My parents graciously offered to let us move in with them while we secured the permits to build our new home. Matt had been packing a storage space in Eastport. We brought boxes of photographs to his mother's dry attic. I also had stored plastic containers filled with possible necessities in my parents' basement for easy access while we lived there.

Matt had a list of builders to interview. We had settled on a house design, but he had ideas for closets, walls, and bathrooms to alter. I had no eye or feel for room dimensions. Matt paced out the perimeters of rooms in the yard so I could "see" the house. There was so much that had to be considered and managed before we could even think of breaking ground, but we projected to be in our brand-new home by June 2008—July at the latest.

chapter thirty-eight

Labor Day

From: Antoinette
To: Colleen
Date: Thursday, August 30, 2007 at 10:15 a.m.
Subject: Labor Day!

I bought tiaras. I got the "Fight Like a Girl" logo on a T-shirt transfer. I will iron them on at home. I have a variety of white tank and T-shirts in a variety of sizes. They are leftovers from projects. What would you like? I will be in Sayville early this afternoon. I want to bring flowers to my mom. Her last living aunt passed away this week. The old lady was a character and had a ball for 93 years, pink hair and all. Mom is taking it hard. I'll give you a call if I'm making good time and maybe drop in on you. In the meantime, have a great day.

Hug everyone you know.
Ann

From: Colleen
To: Antoinette
Date: Thursday, August 30, 2007 at 10:35 a.m.
Subject: Labor Day!

Since I am now "hot" (not the sexy kind, the sweaty kind) 24/7, I would vote on some type of tank top to put over a bathing suit. Let me know if you lay out big bucks, and I'll chip in. I think the boas set me back a whopping $25. I'm headed up to Smithtown this afternoon for a bonding session with my therapist. I will see you on Saturday. Sorry to hear about your aunt, but that's the kind of longevity we want in our gene pools! XXOO

Colleen

Last one! I brought Dr. Sheren and Rose Ann happy sunflowers and mint from the garden and baked ginger cookies for the nurses in the infusion room. This was the last day of chemotherapy, a reason to celebrate. Rose Ann quickly stabbed the port and steadied me as I grew pale. The damn thing still hurt.

"It's flowing well, but I could redo it again," she offered.

I shook my head. Matt concurred; we just wanted to get this done. Dr. Sheren was pleased with my white blood count and that I was having a great summer. The reduced work schedule had helped a great deal, as had the beach time and the signing of a contract to sell the house. As I sipped cold water, we discussed the upcoming port removal (yay!), getting my records to the radiology facility, and setting up a follow-up visit back at Sloan Kettering in November.

Dr. Sheren was not concerned about my thirty-five-pound weight loss since February. Despite this little perk, the scale hovered just under two hundred pounds. I still had plenty of fighting weight. I needed to be committed to this weight loss and truly adopt healthier eating habits. A constant state of nausea was not a good diet plan. I would also need to establish an exercise routine to help keep my body's hormones in balance—especially estrogen. Estrogen was not my friend. It fed the greedy cancer. And although I would be on hormone therapy for five years after the chemo and radiation therapies, estrogen could happily lurk in the body fat, waiting for its chance to strike again. This was going to take a lot of me taking care of me.

The nurses were happy to receive the cookies I baked. I thanked them all for being so patient and wonderful to me and my husband during this time. I added that we were in a rush to catch a ferry to Fire Island when I was done that day. Luckily, the infusion room operated at a quiet hum. I did not complain about the port's burning throb. The treatment went relatively quickly.

When I was unplugged, I hugged each of my nurses. What a blessing to be in such skilled and loving hands! Matt and I practically skipped out the door at four forty-five.

At the car, Matt grabbed me and planted a long, hard kiss on my lips. "You did it!"

"Let's go, big guy," I said, wiping tears from his face. "We have a party to get to!"

Our friends were waiting for us on the Bensons' deck.

Nick had champagne chilling, and he poured glasses while I hugged, kissed, and cried happy tears. We toasted to our health, our wonderful friends, our beautiful bay and beaches, and our love. It was good to be us. I fell asleep early that evening to the sound of the blustery north wind singing through the sailboat shrouds.

The wind howled from the northeast before the dawn. Choppy waves slapped about the shallow cove, straining the anchor lines on the moored boats. I rose early to stretch out the achy bones and joints and set up the drip coffee maker. The full house slept soundly. Only the gurgling coffee maker penetrated the sleepy sighs of the Kovarick family and Matt in the cozy beach house.

I walked to the ocean cupping a large mug of black coffee, no sugar, in my hands. The houses and stunted chokecherry trees blocked the northeast wind so that the ocean lazily tumbled to shore. Beyond the short breakers, the water lay flat with traces of wind currents on the surface far into the clear horizon, giving the illusion of calm seas. I could smell the change of season. Crisp morning breezes heralded the not-so-far-away autumn. Cumulus billows had within days been replaced by wispy cirrus clouds. The sun rose, blindly erasing the red and purple stains from the eastern sky. I gulped the last of the coffee and stretched my arms high, reaching up on my toes to unravel my full length. It promised to be a beautiful day. Time to play!

By noon, the little stretch of sand at the end of Pepperidge Walk was lined with beached Sunfish and small catamarans, their bows facing north toward the mainland. White racing sails and colorful cruising sails, flapping in the wind, decorated the shore. Titus Kana, the Bensons' across-the-boardwalk neighbor, was the master organizer of the Davis Park Labor Day Regatta. For more than twenty years, he had pulled together beach talent and resources to design and produce T-shirts, register participants in the junior and adult races, and manage the official rules and judges. Although strategy was always encouraged, calm respect and sportsmanship toward fellow sailors and paddlers was paramount.

Most of the participants were casual sailors, content to sail in perfect conditions without time or destination constraints. Few had any real racing knowledge or experience. Instead of sailing behind the start line and vying for an advantageous position to start the race within a three-minute countdown, we all stood in the water at the line, holding on to our boats. When the horn blew, we had to jump on, pull the sails in to catch the wind, and take off for the first turn marker. In this way, crashes and false starts were minimized.

The wind continued to blow from the northeast with gusty bursts, creating a skippy chop for the little boats. There were seven Sunfish at the standing start line. Although Sunfish are small boats, a crew was required to race with a skipper in this regatta. This encouraged more people to participate. Dave and Julie Otis had threatened to beat me this year. I had countered that despite their new and much lighter boat and pretty pink-and-yellow sail, I had my ringer: Aileen Kovarick, the "Little Linguini." For the past three years, little Aileen had held the mainsheet tight and leaned her negligible weight on the windward side to balance my boat. She was twelve years old now but remained the thin and strong Little Linguini I counted on.

We took off at the sound of the mini-foghorn, tacking for the windward marker, jibing to a broad reach for the next. The wind blew stiff. A few Sunfish flipped onto their sides, spilling skipper and crew into the bay. I took a chance by sharply rounding the mark but could not recover quickly enough from the jibe. Over we went. Aileen gasped as she plunged into the cold bay.

Luckily, the Sunfish was designed for easy righting. We just needed to weigh down the daggerboard and scramble back onto the hull. Aileen, who proved to be a good swimmer, was a strong girl, but we had to rely on my heft to get the boat righted. I instructed her to hold on to the bow as I pointed the boat into the wind and pulled myself onto the daggerboard. True to form, the boat came up, sails dripping and flapping into the strong wind. Aileen scampered aboard and grabbed the mainsheet. I surprised myself by being able to quickly hoist up onto the boat and steer us back into the race.

By the time the sail filled, the safety boat had come up alongside us.

"Ann, are you okay?" the concerned captain shouted.

"Get out of my way," I shouted back, "I have to catch up!"

Dave and Julie had taken a safer tack around the mark and remained upright. Aileen and I caught up and managed to slip in front of them. Aileen leaned her lithe body over the healing windward side while I tweaked tiller and mainsheet to the maximum advantage. My boom grazed their mast as we sped by. We came in for a third place win, beating Dave and Julie out of a beer mug trophy.

Matt and Nick took out an ancient catamaran with a beer cooler strapped to the mast in the next race. They kept upright through the course, cheering each mark with a beer, and came in third out of four.

Our Pink Power Kostume Kayak splashed in the choppy cove. Matt and Eric, held the boat—meant for three people—steady as Dr. Pam, Lisa, Colleen, and I squeezed ourselves in. Matt duct taped a surgical IV pole onto the side. Ziploc sandwich bags filled with bay water hung from the pole. We taped the tubes to the bags on one end, and to our chests on the other. We wore silly pink hats and tiaras, plastic sunglasses with pink rhinestones, and tank tops with the Fight Like a Girl logo on them. A Pink Power banner ran from bow to stern. There was no room for paddles, let alone balance. When the kayak race horn blew, Matt and Eric held on to our kayak and paraded us along the shore. Mom followed along the beach, wrapped in an electric pink boa, cheering with her pink pom-poms. The men carefully turned us around and safely beached the kayak for a pretend win. We waved to Terry, watching from a relatively germ-free distance on top of the boardwalk. She hailed to us with both arms and her famous broad smile.

What a day! By six thirty, heavy exhaustion pressed down hard. I fell asleep in the Kovaricks' beach house, missing dinner and a spectacular sunset.

From: Antoinette
To: My Everyone
Date: Monday, September 3, 2007 at 7:12 p.m.
Subject: All Done!

Greetings all! Friday was my last chemo treatment! YAHOO!! I went in with home-grown herb bouquets for my doctor and the extremely patient nurse who pokes the port as gently as possible, and a plate of lemon ginger squares for the wonderful nurses in the infusion room. Although happy that this was the very-last-time-ever chemo treatment, I secretly hoped my bribes might get it waived. Matt reminded me that kind of reality only works in my little mind. Oh well, counts were good to go with the treatment. The nurses were very quick in getting us out since we had a ferry to catch to get a start on our Labor Day weekend. Now that chemo is done, I will be arranging radiation therapy that will probably begin in a month or so. I have been warned that the fatigue may be a significant side effect, but I believe that this will be an anxiety-free cakewalk compared to chemo. And besides, who isn't tired?

In two weeks, the port comes out (YIPPEEE!). Although I've been grateful to have it on chemo days, living with it isn't as carefree as the brochures promised. I'll be glad to have the little alien exorcised.

On with Labor Day celebrations. Matt and I bunked in with the Kovaricks. Grateful thanks to Coll and Dan. We participated in the Davis Park Regatta. I sailed my Sunfish with my lightweight, able-bodied crew, Aileen Kovarick, aka "The Little Linguini." Matt sailed with Nick on a TRAC catamaran, and this year my fellow cancer beach bum sisters entered into the Kostume Kayak Kompetition. Mom was our cheerleader! The wind howled, flipping sailboats (mine included), and nearly sank kayaks (Matt and Eric kept our Pink Power kayak steady as we glided in front of the judges). Aileen and I came in a photo finish third place after I almost rammed Dave and Julie Otis out of my way. Matt and Nick took third in their race. But the Pink Power "Fight Like a Girl" Kayak took first place. We represented strength and determination in the face of this hideous disease. We couldn't lose, especially since we pose so pretty in pink!

School begins again. Robyn is settled into routines at the University of Buffalo. Hallie leaves for Chicago soon. As a teacher, early September brings about a sense of renewal and wonderful anticipation. I am so looking forward to my new position at Remsenburg-Speonk. I met fellow teachers and reviewed case files last week. It promises to be a great year.

Thank you all for being a patient ear while I navigated through this odyssey. I couldn't manage this well without the prayers, positive energies, and thoughtful words and love. You are all such a gift. I have to close now. I need to iron my clothes for tomorrow's first day of school. Be well.

Hug everyone you know.
Antoinette

~

From: Renee
To: Antoinette
Date: Monday, September 3, 2007 at 10:32 p.m.
Subject: All Done!

YOU GO GIRL!!!!!! SUPER BIG HUGS

From: Gloria
To: Antoinette
Date: Tuesday, September 4, 2007 at 7:03 a.m.
Subject: All Done!

You must be thrilled. And you're right—radiation can leave you feeling very tired, but at least it is noninvasive! All of my college kids (three of the six) have begun classes. I like your idea of having us cousins go in on a group gift for Aunt Katy and Uncle Phil's fiftieth. Good luck with the new job!

Gloria

part two

Revelations and Tribulations

chapter thirty-nine

New Chapter

School began. I had handed in the last of the signed paperwork to the business office two weeks before. I met Jan Achilich, in her office. I needed to let her know about the cancer treatment and the upcoming radiation therapy.

"Oh, Toni, you look great. You've lost weight!" Jan said when I walked in.

I had to explain that I had not lost the weight with dieting and exercise.

Jan walked around her table and stood in front of me. The blonde pixie powerhouse, immaculately dressed even during the summer, stood barely above my shoulders. She reached up and gave me a big hug. "We are all so happy to have you. There are several of us who have gone through a scare. Some of us have our mothers and sisters battling. You should talk to Linda, our resident survivor."

"Thank you, Jan." I breathed a sigh of relief. "I promise not to let treatment get in the way of my work."

"Do what you need to do. It's important that you stay well," she said.

I left the building that afternoon knowing I had made my best career decision.

I spent the first orientation day meeting new colleagues, signing into the network, and learning the procedures for the school year. Many of the teachers remembered me as a parent. I brought pictures of my girls. I told them I had always believed an important cog in their success could be traced back to the care and attention of these wonderful elementary school teachers.

When my girls passed through Remsenburg-Speonk Elementary School, there were fewer than one hundred children enrolled from kindergarten to sixth grade. Now there were about two hundred kids. Despite the population explosion, the school community remained intimate. Everyone knew everyone. Even the cancer and my impending sale and move were common knowledge.

My caseload was diverse—speech- and language-impaired children as well as a few resource room students. A big chunk of the therapy needs were in kindergarten.

I loved kindergarten. The children were so adorable in their new role as students in the "big school." Learning to be kind, share, play, and follow directions were key to their becoming successful learners and citizens. Reading, math, and writing would eventually make their way into each child's repertoire, but all that knowledge and genius were worthless if a child had never learned to appreciate, respect, and empathize within their community and follow the rules. It was an important social year littered with amazing literature and incredible discoveries, some of which would become embedded into their psyches forever.

Debbie Johnson had been the kindergarten teacher at Remsenburg-Speonk when Robyn began school there. Mrs. Johnson had a patient tone and continually celebrated the endearing qualities of each of her charges—even the most challenging. At the first open school night I attended at Remsenburg-Speonk, she said, "Throughout my very long career, I have taught every elementary grade. I've enjoyed them all, but I am most privileged to teach kindergarten." She smiled at the group of adults sitting in small chairs, knees bent to our ears. She wore a long necklace of little red schoolhouses over her ample breasts. "You can remember back to your kindergarten teacher."

We all nodded at the recall.

"Your child will always remember me," she continued. "I am responsible for making sure your child will have the best possible start to their school life. I strive to be the best kindergarten teacher for your child, worthy of being part of his or her memory."

What a blessing! And now I had the fortune to have this wonderful teacher as a colleague.

The school day was jam-packed. Between planning, implementing, and logging the therapy sessions, coordinating with a team of professionals, and discovering, almost daily, another form to get office materials, pay for a school lunch, or file a work order to fix a sticky doorknob, the school day never ended at 3:40 p.m. I knew it would take time to find a smooth routine. I also knew finding a smooth routine would take a bit longer since I had the port removal surgery and radiation therapy clouding my calendar.

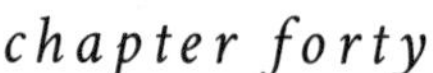

chapter forty

Radiation

I met the radiation oncologist by myself. She flipped through my records as she asked questions, rarely lifting her head from the file as I replied. She concluded that I would have thirty-three consecutive radiation sessions: twenty-seven on the whole breast and the last six aimed directly at the lumpectomy site. I would get tattooed dots to mark the exact areas to aim the radiation at and would need biweekly blood work to ensure that my white blood counts were adequate. I should expect fatigue and skin burns, both of which should be manageable. She did not ask if I had questions, so I volunteered them.

I asked if I should keep the port for further blood testing. She claimed that it would not matter either way since this facility did not draw blood. She preferred that I go to the lab across the street, which would allow her to get the results within a few days. She was not sure if anyone qualified would be available to access the port. Hmmm. I also asked why thirty-three sessions when the radiology oncologist at Memorial Sloan Kettering had figured on a total of twenty-eight.

"That's the way we do it here." She jotted a note in my file.

An uncomfortable moment of silence followed—although it seemed that I was the only one uncomfortable. The radiology oncologist at Memorial Sloan Kettering had gone to great lengths to make sure I had an appreciation for the science of radiation treatments and had said that blood test results there were reported within fifteen minutes. Hmm, again.

I was dismissed to make the appointments for the mapping and tattooing the following week. Although a late afternoon time was not possible for the two one-hour-long sessions, I was assured that the daily treatments could be scheduled at the end of the day.

As I got into my car, my cell phone buzzed. It was the nurse I had just met. The doctor had forgotten to tell me I needed a blood test to rule out pregnancy.

"I am almost fifty, had a tubal ligation eighteen years ago, and have just completed a course of chemotherapy. I am not pregnant."

"This is the way we do things here," the nurse said. "Just come back for the script and get it done within the next few days."

I took a breath, mustered a bit of courage, and said, "I don't think it's necessary. I'll sign whatever waiver is needed. Thank you. Good-bye."

That night I told Matt about the disappointing appointment. He heard the whining creeping into my voice.

Matt sighed. He really wanted—needed—me to be able to do this by myself. Having him juggle his time just to sit in a waiting room for the quick daily treatment sessions was not practical.

"Let's face it," he said, "the Memorial Sloan Kettering experience will be hard to beat, but you need to be reasonable. You have a new job. Hallie is leaving. We are moving. This place is so much closer than Commack and will save you a lot of time and energy. You don't have to love them. You just have to get it done."

I brooded for the rest of the evening. I threw a packed box of linen into the garage, banged the few pans that were left in the kitchen. I was too angry to cry this time. This was supposed to be the easy part of treatment—a cakewalk. Damn it!

But Matt was right. I did not have to love this doctor and her way of doing things. I could, however, refuse the pregnancy test.

chapter forty-one

Port Exorcism

The Rosh Hashanah Jewish holiday gave teachers and students a four-day weekend at the end of September. Pam and Nick offered us their beach house. Matt and I took the ferry to Davis Park on Wednesday night.

Once Labor Day passed, a hush enveloped the beach community. The crowds left for their regular routines, the ferry schedule scaled back, and floating moorings bobbed, untethered, in the cove. Only a handful of retired homeowners happily puttered in their cozy homes during the week.

It was a clear, warm evening. We made it in time to toast the sunset that stained wispy clouds pink and red and reflected orange paths on the still bay. A crisp breeze fluttered the tall cattails. Already the leaves of the chokecherry had begun to fade to crimson and yellow. The autumn equinox would soon push summer into a memory.

I had brought a baked chicken dinner with roasted potatoes and broccoli to warm up. We shared a bottle of wine. That night, with the bay quietly lapping the shore, we lay in bed talking about floor plans, closet space, shower stalls, and ceiling heights. It was all very exciting. Matt could see in his mind's eye exactly how everything would look from every angle. He explained with wide arms and hand gestures the size ratios and layouts he was envisioning. I still needed diagrams and real pictures to see it all, but I nodded, trusting him to make sure my priorities were woven into the plans.

I woke up before dawn. I knew I should spend this quiet time writing lesson plans or, better yet, in my journal. Instead, I stood outside on the deck, overlooking a still bay, as the sun began to lighten to the east. I breathed in my coffee. It smelled magnificent in the beach air. I thought how lucky I was to live in such a beautiful place, to know such wonderful friends, to be born into the best family, and to have a good man by my side. Had I never stopped to contemplate these blessings before?

Matt and I walked to the ocean after breakfast, and he cast a line into the morning ocean. Somehow his sore shoulder did not quake while casting. Surf fishing had been relatively light during the summer. However, since the Labor Day weekend, rumors of striped bass and bluefish near the surf had been keeping fishermen hopeful.

Suddenly, despite the chilly temperature, I had the most incredible hot flash. A full-body, drippy sweat—complete with the panicky need to find cold—erupted. I had been experiencing constant flashes throughout the day, especially when the air temperature was above sixty-eight degrees or after a cup of coffee or glass of wine. This was my body's rebellion against the forced menopause it was being subjected to. Usually, a cold glass of water, stripping down to a tank top, and applying a damp towel were enough to quell the sweating. The trick was to stay calm and keep steady so as not to invite another volley. Occasionally, a flash would grab me so intensely that I truly believed I was melting, like the Wicked Witch in *The Wizard of Oz*. During the summer, I had opened the garden hose on my head, walked into a cool pool, and jumped off a moored boat to keep myself from liquefying into a puddle. This time, I had an ocean in front of me. I quickly surveyed the empty beach, then stripped down to my underwear and leaped past Matt into the surf. Relief!

Matt shook his head and cast in the opposite direction.

The port was scheduled to be removed the next afternoon. Although expecting an anxious day, I was looking forward to getting it out of my chest, out of my consciousness. It had never been comfortable.

We got on the Friday morning ferry back to the mainland. I took two Ativan before walking into ambulatory surgery. The nurse remembered me. I told the surgeon and nurse that I did not want to have the twilight. They both agreed.

The doctor was perplexed that I would not keep the port for a few more months or a year, as most patients do, just to be sure all was clear. I wanted to tell him the port was ugly and uncomfortable—that I felt a sharp pain whenever I leaned over or accidently bumped it. It throbbed when I walked briskly or climbed up and down stairs and was a constant reminder that cancer had infected my life. I wanted to let him know that I only appreciated it for the hour and a half of chemotherapy every three weeks. The rest of the time, it was that alien sticking out of my chest. Instead, I smiled at the friendly doctor and assured him that I did not need it anymore.

Between the Novocaine, Ativan, and squeezing the nurse's

hand, the doctor was able to cut out the port, pull the tube from my neck, and stitch me up within ten minutes, humming to the Four Tops' tune playing over the speakers as he went.

~

From: Antoinette
To: My Everyone
Date: Saturday, September 15, 2007 at 10:29 a.m.
Subject: The Exorcism

YIPPEE! The port is out. I think this is the last of the invasive procedures! I opted for no anesthesia because what they could offer me only puts me into a tailspin of agitation. Novocaine, Ativan, and squeezing the nurse's hand made me a better—well —more manageable patient. I just have to deal with the yucky stitches for a few days.

Matt and I were able to spend Wednesday night and Thursday at the beach, thanks to our best Benson friends. September on the beach is absolutely gorgeous. There is a magical regeneration of spirit that happens with salt air, sand, and the constant sound of the surf.

Our Hallie left for her new life adventure in Chicago. Chicago will be a fun city to visit, especially when Southwest Airlines offers $39 fares—can't afford to stay home.

We continue to pack. It's amazing what fourteen years of living in one place can accumulate. I even found boxes from our old house . . . still unpacked! There will be a BIG garage sale next Saturday in an effort to purge stuff from our lives and storage spots. Please come by to sift through the cra . . . ah . . . treasures.

Take good care of yourselves.

Hug everyone you know.
Antoinette

~

From: Dan and Coll
To: Antoinette
Date: Saturday, September 15, 2007 at 4:43 p.m.
Subject: The Exorcism

Great news! Almost done.

Coll

~

From: Sara
To: Mom
Date: Saturday, September 15, 2007 at 11:21 p.m.
Subject: The Exorcism

Yeah! I hated to look at that thing. Love you,

Sara

~

From: Colleen
To: News from the Back Deck Fans
Date: Tuesday, September 18, 2007 at 5:13 p.m.
Subject: News from the Back Deck

I received a message on my cell phone on my way home from Sloan today. I didn't expect results for a few days! IT'S GOOD NEWS . . . THE TREATMENT IS WORKING . . . THERE IS

NO REMARKABLE INCREASE IN THE SIZE OF THE TUMORS AND SOME HAVE EVEN DECREASED IN SIZE.

Thank you for all of your prayers, hope, and encouragement . . . this proves my theory . . . beach therapy and prayer truly does work!!!!!!!!!!!!!!!! I love you all.

Colleen

What great news for Colleen! Finally hope and a glimmer of possibilities, perhaps a miracle, seemed possible.

chapter forty-two

Radiation and Humiliation

I had to take a half day from work to get scanning and mapping completed. I met two of the technicians, both men, who measured my torso and breast from what seemed to be every angle. I traveled bare-breasted through the CT scan. The only adornment I was allowed was the bandage covering the not-quite-melted stitches from the port site. The technicians talked around me in the way rude cashiers talk over their stations. As I rolled out of the CT ring, another technician had me hold up a plaque with my identification and whatever else they needed over my chest for a photograph. I had never been so publicly uncovered. I'd birthed three large babies with more drapery.

The doctor strolled into the now very crowded CT room, confirming readings. As she left the room, she asked how I was doing. She did not stay long enough for me to answer. It was a long, humiliating hour.

I had always been very self-conscious about my body. I used private stalls to change in gyms, and I never paraded around in my underwear like my suitemates in college. Even in my skinny younger years, I wore cover-ups over bikinis. I was fully aware of my large frame and lumbering grace. Only Matt appreciated my full naked figure—and modesty.

I left with a start date penned in my pocket calendar, appointments for the first week, and a damn prescription for a pregnancy test. I held all emotions and tears in check until I buckled myself into my car. There, I cried out my frustration at having to be so exposed, my ineptitude in not protesting, my outrage over the lack of decency and politeness, and just the pure anger I felt at having to deal with this fucking disease. It was a good, hard cry.

Finally calmed down, I took out a red marker and the datebook from my pocketbook. I counted thirty-three days from the start date and circled November 9. Even if I missed a day or if their equipment broke down for a week, I vowed not to make up the time. I would be absolutely done on November 9—no matter what! I found the prescription for the pregnancy test crumbled in my left hand. Before pulling out of the parking lot, I did something I never did; I threw the wad out of the window.

A few days after the CAT-scan mapping, I had to go in for the tattooing. The tattoo dots would serve as permanent waypoints to line up my body for the radiation zapping. All this prep work aimed to make sure the radiation was only directed at specific sites.

I'd never had a tattoo, nor desired one. Enduring pricks and deep pinches just to draw on my skin seemed barbaric (as compared to the shells and starfish I drew on my teenage legs with a ballpoint pen so many years ago). Perhaps it was a generational rite of passage; tattoos were certainly everywhere. My daughters, especially Sara, were fans, seeing them as a form of self-expression and beauty. The palette of colors and the details artists now offered tempted even those who only occasionally entertained the idea of getting a tattoo.

I was not one of those people. Besides the pain involved, I didn't think I had the long-term attention span for such a permanent adornment. I quickly forgot once-loved jewelry and accessories. Living with a forever tattoo seemed to be an excessive commitment. I also had seen many fallen, stretched, and wrinkled tattoos that had not held up over time. Not pretty.

The radiation tattoos were stabbed into me while I lay, once again, on my back, right breast exposed. On my way out, I reminded the receptionist that I needed late afternoon appointments. She assured me there was no problem with that because she took arrangements into the early evening. She handed me the list of appointments for the remainder of the week—all set.

The cold tone of the radiation team did not warm during those first three radiation sessions. I rushed to the facility as soon as school was dismissed, hoping I had packed all my homework in order to prepare for the next day. There was no waiting. I appeared to be the last patient of the day. The pretty young technician who sat next to the smiling receptionist let out an exasperated sigh when I walked in for that first treatment.

"Am I late?" I asked the receptionist.

"Not at all," she said. She seemed embarrassed. I would have been if a colleague had displayed that kind of disrespect in front of me, too.

I was directed to change into an examination gown, then led to the treatment room, and finally guided to lie flat on the hard table. I was buckled down. The room was cool and thick with padded quiet. The darkness was illuminated only by pin-sized colored lights and monitors, giving the space an eerie aura. The table was elevated, and for at least five full minutes my back, sides, and breasts were pushed, shoved, and slid so the tattoo dots were lined up with the tiny red light beams. The young tech umphed and sighed as the older technician coached her through. Every few pulls and tugs, he brought his face down close to my body, eyeballing the lineup. I was told not to move, not to help, to lie still. I felt like a slab of meat.

Finally, the gun that shoots out the invisible radiation was aimed perfectly, and the technicians scattered to stand safely behind leaded walls. Within a few minutes, I was released from the table. I quickly dressed and scurried out of the building to my car's safe haven. I dug into my pocketbook, pulled out the datebook, and drew a thick red *X* on the day. One down, thirty-two to go.

I could not put off the blood test any longer. On Thursday, I went across the street from the radiation facility to the lab. The phlebotomist was exceptionally compassionate, letting me lie down rather than trying to sit up through a faint. She was quick and accurate. When she finished, I just needed a minute to clear my head before I left. She told me the doctor would probably get results by Tuesday or Wednesday—which meant that if there was a problem, I would have had three or four more treatments before the report came in. Yet another score for this facility being the wrong choice.

~

From: Antoinette
To: My Everyone
Date: Friday, September 28, 2007 at 5:13 p.m.
Subject: Part II

Hello, good friends. Now that chemo is over and forever done with and the port is out, I am getting the radiation therapy portion of treatment complete. Since this part of the protocol is daily, I needed to find a more convenient local site. I will be going to a facility close to work and home. I learned that there will be 33 sessions, every weekday (for about 6-1/2 weeks). I also learned that I am to have biweekly blood work . . . BUT since the office does not draw blood, I have to go to a lab. Anyway, a stick is a stick; I'm never happy, but I will just get it over with. Who knew I would ever get this brave? I was mapped and tattooed last week. The tattoos look as if I was stabbed by a pencil. I can't understand the appeal of tattoos when the four little pricks really hurt!One would have to be contentedly drunk to manage a full picture. Oh! I get it now.

Three sessions were complete this week. It's fine, no pain, and now that we have had some practice, it takes about fifteen minutes. It's just old-fashioned embarrassment, laying on my back, right boob exposed, getting pulled and shoved into position by a man-tech and a young woman tech who rolls her eyes and sighs impatiently. Thirty to go!

In the meantime, Matt and I are diligently packing and preparing to move out. We had a rather successful garage sale last weekend, but the garage is still full of cra—err treasures! Center Moriches Historical Society is coming tomorrow to hopefully take more away. Another dumpster comes next week! We are shooting for a November 5th closing date. Matt went to Islip town today and applied for the necessary permits and tax assessment to start the building process. He was surprised to have a pleasant experience with helpful and efficient clerks. We think we have most of the logistics for moving worked out. I do have one big concern . . . my cat, Willow. My parents have a princess cat who rules the roost. Willow is not friendly. She barely puts up with Petie. It is truly the "Garfield and Odie" show. She would not be happy or safe in a home with other pets. She is affectionate towards anyone who feeds her and is rather self-sufficient, very clean—a very good cat. Does anyone know of a home that is petless and can take Willow until next summer?

In a few weeks, we will start moving into my parents' house. Our Remsenburg phone number will be disconnected, but the cell phone numbers will remain the same. Keep well, my friends.

Hug everyone you know.
Antoinette

~

From: Julie
To: Antoinette
Date: Friday, September 28, 2007 at 6:27 p.m.
Subject: Part II

All sounds like it's going OK. You're on the home stretch! My mom sailed through the daily radiation, so I'm hoping the same for you. I guess a little daily humiliation builds character?! Thinking of you with love,

Julie

~

From: Sherry
To: Antoinette
Date: Saturday, September 29, 2007 at 11:42 a.m.
Subject: Part II

Life is good when we move on. About halfway through the radiation the "chemo fog" lifted, and I can't tell you how great that was! My hair is short but a reasonable length. I was told that I could color it—thank goodness because it was white! Did I ever mention that we were in the midst of a home expansion project during this ordeal? We ended up getting our living room furniture on the last day of my radiation treatments. Good luck with the home move. Keep in touch.

Sherry

~

From: Sara
To: Mom
Date: Saturday, September 29, 2007 at 11:38 p.m.
Subject: Part II

Wow . . . no more 325 phone number! And Mom, you can't be drunk when you get tattooed because it thins your blood and makes a mess! Cheers.

Sara

From: Robyn
To: Mom
Date: Sunday, September 30, 2007 at 1:43 a.m.
Subject: Part II

Don't give Willow away! I'll take her if I can get an apartment next semester.

Robyn
OH, and I love you.

chapter forty-three

Birthday Blues

Hallie and Robyn are exactly three years and eight hours apart in age. It was not planned. Sara and Hallie were born within a week of their projected due dates. When Robyn's expected date of delivery was targeted for Hallie's actual birthday, I did not think it could be possible. Who had a baby on her due date? But Robyn insisted on her debut being October 5. A few days before, my mom and sisters helped me put together a family birthday party for Hallie. We blew out candles, ate chocolate cake, and ripped birthday wrapping paper and ribbons to reveal new favorite frilly dresses and Gumby and Pokey toys. A baby sister arriving on Hallie's birthdate was the bonus.

I loved the idea of star twins. I envisioned the sisters growing into similar people with matching skills and temperaments. The stars—well, at least the dates—were lined up. I soon learned that there was nothing cosmic about siblings being born on the same day.

"Siblings sharing a birthdate happens all the time, more often than actual twins," our pediatrician said while examining newborn Robyn. The nurse, recording vitals, confirmed with a nod.

"In fact," the doctor continued, "many family members' birthdays are within a few weeks, even days of each other."

I still loved the idea of star twins. Although we ate too much cake during the first week of October and I scrambled to pull off celebrations that gave both Hallie and Robyn a sense of individual specialness, I enjoyed the uniqueness, even if it was a frequent occurrence.

Hallie and Robyn, of course, did not grow to have similar temperaments, skills, or interests. In fact, all three of my girls grew into very different young women: Sara, always focused, driven, and incredibly creative; Hallie, sensitive, sweet, and gifted in the spoken and written word; Robyn, daring and adventurous, always looking for a way to explore Earth's beauty. Their differences steered their young adult selves into varying career paths and relationships.

The girls also did not look like each other the way most sisters do. My sisters' daughters strongly resembled their mother—in their facial features, hair, and body build. They looked as if they belonged to each other, with their mother at the apex. My girls, meanwhile, seemed to have taken the best of Matt and me to come up with three different looks. Sara had my tight curls and deep brown eyes and Matt's weak chin (perfect aperture for the clarinet). Hallie's thick, wavy hair and light coloring came from her father, but she inherited a beautiful profile and her broad smile from the Truglio side of the family. Robyn's long, lean body was similar to mine, and her thick, straight chestnut hair (the hair I'd always wanted) was akin to my sister Diana's, but her fair complexion was her dad's.

Although each daughter branched off from the parental tree trunk with their own physical features, personalities, and quirks, each shared a surname, spoke with similar voice patterns, used similar body gestures, held an intense work ethic, and was deeply devoted to her sisters and our family. Perhaps this was enough to glue together the sisterhood—much more so than a date on the calendar.

This year, Hallie and Robyn were scattered. I ached with missing them on their star twin birthday. Sending a gift via Amazon and leaving a singing message on their voicemail felt like an empty gesture.

My brother, Bill, came over with a truck and moved the piano to his home. I hoped my young nieces would appreciate piano lessons and enjoy playing more than my girls had. I had bought the piano some ten years before from the music store where the girls were taking clarinet and guitar lessons. It was refurbished and had a wonderful timbre. The lemon-oil smell of the keys and wood brought me back to my grandmother's Brooklyn flat. The apartment had held tight living quarters for my father's extended family, but even so my grandfather's baby grand piano had sat tucked into a dining room corner, filling precious space with music and joy.

My dad brought that piano to his much larger house when Grandma moved to the suburbs to be closer to her charges. I was sixteen or seventeen—too old for lessons. As a child, Dad had taken lessons but as an adult played mostly by ear and memory. He claimed never to have had the talent and passion his father had as a musician. As far as my own daughters were concerned, Robyn did not stick to the lessons. Sara occasionally picked out tunes. I hoped that I might take lessons one day, but it never happened. There was always something else to do.

A POD was delivered to the driveway. Friends with strong backs helped us pack the 10x15 container with furniture that might fit in the new house. A POD usually sits in a driveway for a few weeks while home renovation projects ensue, but since we needed a longer window of time, we had decided to have our filled POD stored in an old hangar in Calverton.

I worked on changing our address. I picked up the paperwork at the Remsenburg post office, then drove out to Sayville to rent a PO Box. I also settled the fate of the pets during our home building interim. Petie would live in foster care at Helga and Carla's. He was happy in their home with a fenced yard to guard over, and we could easily visit him. Mom, meanwhile, agreed to let my cranky cat live upstairs while her skittish cat reigned downstairs.

The lists in my head continued to loop. I constantly cross-referenced my date book, the home calendar hanging on the refrigerator, the to-do lists scribbled on notepaper that were scattered on tables, counters, stuffed into my pocketbook. I felt that something was missing. What was I forgetting?

The chemo fog had yet to lift. It had been over a month

since the last hit, and yet I remained slow-witted and insecure in thinking and juggling my way through my days. Food smells and tastes were still not right in my nose and belly. I really missed chocolate—just a whiff still triggered a metallic taste that sat in my mouth for hours. I expected a lack of energy but had hoped that food would start tasting better while I was undergoing radiation. Would this be the new me? The radiation oncologist had no information for me regarding that complaint.

Matt's lists were no less cluttered. He had detailed plans ready for an architect, and even more 3-D details playing out in his head. His paper and computer renderings continued to be lost on me. He still paced out the closet spaces and bathrooms for me to "see." But I noticed that his pace in obtaining necessary county and town permits had slowed. The general contractor search had also stalled, and the piles of papers on the dining room table remained untouched. It had been a while since he'd rolled out the prints to talk about another idea, another feature.

Finally, he admitted his apprehension.

"I just want to be sure the house actually sells," he said. "It's been hard enough buying the property without selling the house. I don't want to sink any more money into something that may not happen."

My heart sank. "Did you hear something? Did the realtor say anything?"

"No," he said, "but with the economy tanking, the buyers being overseas and paying cash . . . I won't trust this whole thing until the money gets into the bank."

Throughout our twenty-eight-year marriage, I had orchestrated a handful of crazy exploits (like taking a three-year-old and an infant on a bareboat charter to the Caribbean). It was my idea to get a runabout motorboat for the girls instead of a car, and to buy the handyman special in Remsenburg and fix it up enough to rent it so we could live at Davis Park each summer. I also came up with the plot to purchase the property in Sayville from Matt's sisters, sell our Remsenburg place, and build a house—a project Matt had always wanted to tackle.

Although Matt liked my big ideas, he was the one who had to work out the practical logistics. If we did not have each other, I would have run my inattentive and impulsive self into financial and social ruin, and he would have led a boring and predictable life.

~

From: Dr. Pam
To: Antoinette
Date: Sunday, October 7, 2007 at 5:16 p.m.
Subject: Pam's update

It's me (Greg), using Pam's e-mail account. I thought you might appreciate a quick update on how Pam is doing. As you know, shortly after the first chemo treatment, Pam lost all of her hair. Despite this, she kept her sense of humor. We recently attended her partner's birthday party. Pam wore her wig for the first time (she usually wears her "do-rags"). She got a big hug from one of the retired partners in her practice that nearly knocked it off her head. We were in the reception area of the country club wetting our pants laughing as I helped her straighten out the crooked hairpiece on her head. Plainly, she is keeping her good spirits and does not miss a beat. In fact, I cannot remember the last time that Pam had a "pity party" for herself (whereas I can think of hundreds that I have had myself). She is amazing. Throughout all of this, Pam has continued to work full-time "birthin' babies," taking "calls," and holding office hours. The hardest part about working is that she has to constantly tell the story to her patients. Many end up crying on the exam table, and Pam ends up comforting them! While she never complains, I know that she is very weary of this whole "cancer thing."

In any event, we are now moving on to the next phase of her treatment. On Wednesday, October 24, Pam will undergo a bilateral mastectomy at the Chester County Hospital. During the same surgery, the reconstruction process will begin, with the placement of "tissue expanders" under her pectoral muscles. After a couple of months, she will have another outpatient surgical procedure to have the tissue expanders removed and the implants inserted. There will be a couple of minor procedures after that (and taking the drug Tamoxifen for five years), but she will be done. We hope to start 2008 cancer free. Thanks, as always, for your thoughts, prayers, cards, meals, and generosity. While this may sound cliché, Pam has gained a great deal of strength and courage from the support of all of you. Please stay in touch, and I will give you an update after her surgery on the 24th.

Greg

Jeez! Just when I thought I deserved to sink into a pity party for myself, I get Greg's e-mail. Dr. Pam had shown so much courage through her chemotherapy, and now she continued to do so in the face of the upcoming mastectomy and reconstruction surgeries. I could not imagine going through all that invasion, working long, grueling hours taking care of others, and then coming home to care for her very busy young family.

Dr. Pam and I shared a common aim: get through whatever had to be done, take care of our families, work hard at our jobs, and remain focused on the prize—a long, healthy life. I printed Greg's e-mail and kept it in my datebook as a reminder.

❋

chapter forty-four

Re-Fitting a New Me

Aunt Kay had been planning her and Uncle Phil's fiftieth anniversary celebration, complete with flowers, place settings, dinner, and dancing to a doo-wop band, for months. She wanted everyone to attend. "Everyone" included siblings, cousins, nieces, nephews, and their families, as well as close friends who were considered family.

Aunt Kay had called me after my last chemo treatment.

"I want to be sure you will be there, Antoinette," she said. "You and your mother missed my wedding because you were born just two days before. You can't miss this party."

My cousins, aunts, and uncles had been constants throughout my life. They were always present for celebrations, holidays, Sundays, outings, and adventures. My extended family was truly a family that knew each other well and looked forward to visits and events. Aunt Kay, my father's sister, and Uncle Phil's family were especially close given that we shared boating and fishing escapades. How they had managed all of the kids running, crawling, climbing, and falling without losing one over the years was a marvel. Aunt Kay and Uncle

Phil were my parents' best friends—their kids my first playmates. My happiest childhood memories included them. There was no way I would miss this party.

"I will definitely be there, Aunt Kay," I assured her. "I am fine."

The bathroom scale proclaimed a fifty-two-pound weight loss since January. WOW! Who knew that shedding pounds would be a breast cancer perk? I shopped online to buy new slacks and blouses for work. I needed a fancy dress for the anniversary party and had no idea what would look good on my deflated body. I had to go to a store.

I did not like to shop. I avoided malls. There was no joy in browsing through racks, dressing and undressing in fitting rooms, inspecting angles in mirrored walls, pretending my legs looked better without ankle socks. Online shopping always worked well for me because it was pressure-free. My arm and leg length were true to standard sizes, and my fashion sense remained simple and practical.

For this party, however, I wanted to look better than good. My fiftieth birthday was approaching. I had recently had the uneven wisps and the thinned patches on my crown shaped by a stylist to disguise the chemotherapy side effects. The hair sheddings I'd experienced throughout treatment had resulted in a manageable mane—another breast cancer perk. The hair color from the box was very close to my natural dark brown color. But the haircut and color were not nearly enough. I wanted my family to see me healthy, even pretty. I had to go to a store for a dress.

I knew I did not want a friend, mother, or sister with me on this shopping trip. It only made me more impatient when someone who thought shopping was fun suggested more items to try on and more stores to explore. I went alone to Dress Barn.

The store had a few customers milling about. A saleswoman directed me to the party dresses. All I knew was that I wanted a mid-length dress that was not black. She suggested a few styles, and within five minutes she had an armful of dresses for me to try on in an array of sizes.

The second dress, size ten, slipped on, zipped up easily, and glittered with green rhinestones. I would never have entertained a dress like this a year ago. It was a strapless emerald green with a sparkling black webbing pattern on the skirt. The black shrug jacket hid the port scar. The dress fell to mid-calf, with just the right amount of black tooling peeking from the hem.

"Beautiful," the saleswoman said. A customer struggling into a pencil skirt exclaimed, "Wow!"

I didn't remember ever having gotten a "wow!" compliment before. Ever. I raised my arms in front of the mirror and announced, "Sold!"

The saleswoman talked me into a lovely green necklace to go with the dress. Within a half hour of walking into the store, I was out the door, carrying my prizes in a plastic garment bag. I would worry about shoes and a strapless bra later. For now, I had a dress worthy of a celebration.

From: Antoinette
To: My Sisters, Brother, & Cousins
Date: Tuesday, October 9, 2007 at 8:10 p.m.
Subject: Anniversary Party

How is everyone? Matt and I have been busy with the sale of the house, the move (another Dumpster is coming), and this pesky cancer business. I've been collecting your suggestions for a group gift for Aunt Kay and Uncle Phil from us—their nieces and nephews. How about a donation in their name to the Ronald McDonald House? Aunt Kay was always happy to hear of the good work this foundation had done, especially for Diana's Sandy. I will be sending details soon on how to contribute. Be well, everyone. Can't wait to see all of you at the party.

Hug everyone you know.
Antoinette

~

From: Barbara
To: Antoinette
Date: Tuesday, October 9, 2007 at 8:58 p.m.
Subject: Anniversary Party

Wow—everything at once—radiation, move, so much. I hope you are hanging in there and remembering to smile each day. I think I need a Dumpster, too, since I am trying to get rid of stuff. It's been very hard sifting through the remnants of this marriage. I love the gift idea. I think it is right on. So who is bringing kids, and who is going alone? Aunt Kay put "Barbara and Guest" on the invite, but I am wondering if it will be too much for everyone to see me there with someone. Diana is still not talking to me. I don't know what she is so very bent about. So I will just call and beg her forgiveness for anything and everything since it just is not worth going to the party and through the holidays like this. I really have enough tension in my life—I don't need more. Miss you.

Barbara

~

Sisters. It's amazing how different the four of us are from each other, considering we came from the same parents and were raised in the same home and schools and with seemingly the same set of expectations.

Three years and eleven months separate me and my youngest sister, Barbara. Mary and Diana were plopped in between. Bill arrived a little more than two years after Barbara. My earliest memories feature a round mommy with a long, bouncy ponytail and red lipstick outlining lullabies, demands, and kisses. Despite the short amount of time that passed between each of our births, we all went on to take varying side streets into life, creating our own version of family and place in the world.

And yet we have always been pulled toward each other. There is a true force of attraction, a real need to be included, to include them and their burdens, accept whatever comes by, allow forgiveness to heal wounds. We value those ties. It goes beyond the blood. My sisters have known me from the beginning, and they may be the only ones with me in the end. Through all our differences, through all our varying opinions on almost every subject, we remain sisters. True blessings.

Barbara was having a very rough year. When her husband of nearly twenty years left her, she found herself alone with two teenage girls, complete with adolescent challenges, a cluttered house, and the sense of being thrown away. My heart broke for her. I worried about her choice of men now that she was dating, her girls' adjustments to their parents' choices, and how she would navigate her way through the divorce.

Although I had offered my shoulder whenever Barbara called or visited, it was Diana—closest in age, her home and college roommate, and the sister with daughters the same age as her daughters—whom she'd wanted and needed most over the past year. But there was some kind of argument between them that had sparked this latest standoff. I heard Diana's venting and one-sided versions and saw Barbara shrugging off her points, but I didn't fully understand the heart of the problem. Truth be told, I did not have the energy to mediate the issues—and besides, no one asked me to. Diana's grip on grudges and trespasses were not lost on Barbara. It was so much easier to ask for absolution and get on with the everyday. Life was too short for anger and blame.

chapter forty-five

The Green Slide

After two weeks of radiation therapy, the atmosphere at the radiation facility remained cold and frustrating. I almost sprinted out of the building to the safety of my car after each treatment, humiliated by the exposure and my failure to speak up for myself. Through angry tears, I crossed out the date and recounted how many more days until November 9.

To top off my bad mood, skin burns appeared. It was bad enough that the affected breast was now noticeably smaller and stared off to the right. It now sported a dark purple color and open sores. So much for my theory that my Mediterranean skin would handle the radiation zappings.

The doctor recommended a lotion, but when I tried it I found that it left anything it touched greasy and odorous. Since chemotherapy, the lightest scents and most minimal of textures could result in waves of nausea crashing through my body. The doctor shrugged as she left the room, saying the cream was the best on the market.

Hallie suggested aloe gel from the health food store to

minimize burn damage. Clean, unscented aloe gel did not contain synthetic processing. She had worked in a health food store during her college years and effortlessly navigated the aisles, expounding on the benefits of soy blocks, rice milk, and tree barks as we walked past the shelves that held them. She enjoyed talking the talk with the clerks, comparing the latest and greatest benefits of a Himalayan flower or jellyfish tentacle.

Before cancer hit home, I had dabbled in the ways of the green side. I appreciated the value of organic produce and free-range meats. I searched for and tasted colorful roots and gritty grains that challenged my culinary skills and offered my family healthy variety. However, reading and sifting through the theory and practice of herbal products quickly exhausted my patience. It was difficult to digest the confident yet unsupported narratives they offered.

Still, I had always been intrigued by these products' claims that they might do something about those elusive free radicals, improve short-term memory, or strengthen fingernails. I occasionally went to the local health food shop only to find myself glazing over at first contact with unpronounceable supplements and unproven promises. Inevitably, I returned to my familiar grocery store to buy chewable vitamins and frozen blueberries.

Dr. Sheren advised me not to take extra steps toward health improvement during treatment because the supplements might contraindicate the principle purpose of poisoning the cancer. I was quietly relieved to have that burden lifted but disappointed that I would not be in control of yet another variable concerning my body as I battled the disease.

Hallie sent me a list of instructions on what to look for (and look out for) in an aloe gel. She called from Chicago to deliver a motivating pep talk for the next day's excursion. I set out armed and ready to take back some control.

The tight aisles were crammed ten feet high with remedies for every type of bite, bump, or burp you could imagine. After I had browsed through gels that managed everything from bee stings to colon repair, a young, braless clerk in a sweeping biodegradable dress and hemp sandals adorning dirty feet offered to help. I was intrigued by her blonde Rastafarian hair and thick eyebrows. She immediately expressed an audible gasp upon learning that I had recently finished six months of chemotherapy and was now undergoing radiation therapy.

"Ahh! You should have come in sooner," she said, shaking her head. "It will take years to purge the pollutants from your body and soul."

I was tempted to confront her on this point. After all the research I had plunged into to decide on the most successful and aggressive treatment options for my type of breast cancer, I knew what I was doing. My goal was to never face cancer ever again. I wanted her to know that my mother and grandmother, as well as thousands of fellow sisters, had pioneered before me and endured trial protocols, making survival more possible and safer for me and the next generation of newly diagnosed. If she had real proof that green leafy vegetables cured cancer, she would have to wash her feet and get to the nearest hospital with the word *CANCER* sprawled across them!

But I was there to buy aloe gel, not start a debate. Life is too short to get angry at people who have not walked in my shoes.

"I'll start with the gel," I replied.

She claimed that the chosen gel was as pure as possible but would not keep my skin and general health in good balance. She went on about how I was to love myself (not enough self-love causes cancer?) and began what looked like a self-massage routine in the tight aisle. Yikes! Abandoning Hallie's list, I quickly bought the small tube and darted for the door.

I wanted to learn the ways of the green side. Hallie said she would put together a "dummies" version of information—something in Mom-ese that would give me courage. I promised myself that when this cancer treatment is behind me, I will venture through those aisles again. I may have to find another shop, though.

The aloe gel did soothe the angry sores with its cool magic. It also felt good to take back a little control.

~

From: Antoinette
To: My Everyone
Date: Friday, October 12, 2007 at 7:50 p.m.
Subject: Hello Friends

Hello, good friends and family. I am two weeks into the radiation treatments. Although there is no pain, vein stabbings, or mind-fogging side effects, the daily trip for the ten-minute R&H session (radiation and humiliation) to Riverhead is grinding. I am also disappointed that this facility is not as streamlined, user-friendly, or communicative as

Sloan. I'm feeling stuck. Now my skin has some very ugly burns. Hallie suggested aloe gel from the earth and twig shop in town. A young, braless clerk offered to help. When I told her I had just finished chemotherapy and now had radiation burns, she stated that I should have come in when I was first diagnosed. She finally suggested a gel, but, alas, it would not keep my skin and health in good balance. She went on about how I was to love myself and started to demonstrate a massage routine on herself. I quickly bought the gel before she came to a climax!

Matt and I continue to pack and slowly move into my parents' house. We have a closing date: November 5! Matt has a good feeling about a builder and architect. 2008 is looking great. Enjoy the autumn, now that it is finally here!
Keep well.

Hug everyone you know.
Antoinette

~

From: Hallie
To: Mommy
Date: Friday, October 12, 2007 at 11:15 p.m.
Subject: Hello Friends

I am not sure how to respond, but I'm glad you got what you need. Stay tough, Mommy.

~

From: Sherry
To: Antoinette
Date: Saturday, October 13, 2007 at 7:23 a.m.
Subject: Hello Friends

November 9 is right around the corner! I just had my PET/CT scan and it was clear of any cancer. YAHOO!!!!!!!!!! It's been a year now, and I feel that I am truly on the mend!

~

From: Antoinette
To: Sherry
Date: Saturday, October 13, 2007 at 1:25 p.m.
Subject: Hello Friends

Such great news for you, Sherry! Now to get strong. Keep well, my friend.

~

From: Lisa
To: Antoinette
Date: Saturday, October 13, 2007 at 11:48 a.m.
Subject: Hello Friends

Girl, don't get me started on my well-meaning but useless, misguided "organic" friends! While going through one of my treatments, I got to talking to the girl having chemo next to me. She thought she could self-contain her tumor "naturally" when she was first diagnosed. Now she is trying to contain an aggressive advancing tumor the old-fashioned way—with six rounds of chemo and a higher staging. I do try to mind what I eat, but these people just make me want to munch Big Macs.

Phew—sorry to vent there. It just burns me up when people talk about things so authoritatively because they "once saw an article somewhere . . ." November 9 is just around the corner. You are so close.

Lisa xxx

chapter forty-six

More Birthday Blahs

From: Barbara
To: Antoinette
Date: Thursday, October 18, 2007 at 5:57 p.m.
Subject: Happy Birthday

Happy birthday to you,
Happy birthday to you,
Happy birthday dear Auntie Ann,
Happy birthday to you.

XXOO Barbara, Angela, & Brianna

~

From: Antoinette
To: Barbara
Date: Thursday, October 18, 2007 at 6:57 p.m.
Subject: BLAH Birthday

Thank you, but I am ignoring this sucky year. I want a do-over.

Hug Everyone You Know

Dad never tolerated the word *hate*. "It is such an ugly word," he preached to his young children. "It has no place in my home with my beautiful family." I learned to save such a horrible word for special occasions.

I tried my dad's line on my adolescent daughters when they slammed doors, proclaiming a hatred for their sisters, their homework, macaroni, me—but somehow my delivery was not as powerful as my dad's, because they never held back on expressing their feelings.

This radiation treatment had brought the word to a higher level for me. I absolutely hated it. I hated walking into the office. I hated having to undress, lie down on the hard table, be shoved and pulled into position, then zapped. I especially hated the morose young technician who sauntered back into the room to swing the gun away and unstrap me, sighing and seeming so put out by doing her job. The hatred grew especially strong for the cold doctor. *Hate.* It was becoming a more regular part of my vocabulary.

I'd always kept my birthday low-key. I was not someone who wanted everyone wishing me a great day all day or to have anyone feel obligated to do anything special. I appreciated my girls acknowledging the day with a call, a small gift. Mom always had a lovely card for me with a sentimental message and a check—enough to go out to a nice dinner with Matt (I got my don't-like-to-shop genes from her). For several years, Matt cooked and tried to clean up after preparing tomatoes stuffed with lobster salad—my favorite. He prided himself on pulling the lobster out himself—a chore he really did not like—and choosing the best of the last tomatoes in our garden.

But it was my fiftieth birthday, and I did not want any of it. It was hard enough to turn the corner on half a century, start receiving AARP programs addressed to me, and officially become part of the middle-aged census. I felt ugly, frustrated, and anxious on this birthday. The constant hot-flashing stopped me midstride at all hours. I cried over the smallest obstacle, unable to articulate what had triggered the floods. The most trivial thought made me duck under a wad of tissues. I would happily turn fifty next year.

Matt, however, was not going to chance me being serious about letting my birthday slide. When I arrived at school the day of, a gorgeous bouquet of my favorite pink and red roses—arranged in a slender vase with the most complicated shimmering pink bow cascading down the sides—awaited me in the school's front office. Word got around quickly. During my lunch break, I was greeted with sincere birthday congratulations. As I uncovered my salad, a young teacher came up behind me and placed his hands on my shoulder. I turned to his sweet smile. "All the best of the day to you, Toni," he said.

I pushed my salad away and cried into my folded arms. Poor guy.

Right after school, I drove home and placed my roses on the counter. I had canceled the radiation appointment earlier in the day—*screw* being a compliant do-gooder. I put Petie in his sweater and harness and drove the two of us to Roger's Beach, an oceanfront strip of beach in Westhampton.

We never bothered with town during the summer. The Hamptons spilled over with people; shops, restaurants, and beaches were all far too crowded. Besides, we had to buy a beach permit to park at the beaches. The money was better spent on boat dockage. In October, though, the crowds moved back to the city, the town regained its quiet composure, and the fee collectors at the beach pavilions returned to college.

The beach sprawled wide and infinite. Petie and I walked along the sand, watching sandpipers grazing on the shore and enjoying the warm breeze, clear, endless skies, and comforting constant of the surf. This was much better than enduring a radiation treatment on my birthday. I let Petie off the leash. He marked every seaweed patch in our path while I aimlessly sifted through sand for beach glass and intact scallop shells. We took a long, careless walk, which was a feat since I had limited endurance and Petie's heart remained enlarged and inefficient.

I pulled into the driveway just as Matt was taking grocery bags from his car. He was surprised to see Petie leap from my car and jump up to his hip height with exuberant joy.

"What happened?" he asked.

"Petie and I walked the beach. I canceled radiation."

He nodded as he opened the front door. "Good idea."

"And I'm not making up the treatment session."

"Oh. Okay."

From: Antoinette
To: My Everyone
Date: Friday, October 19, 2007 at 1:52 p.m.
Subject: Birthday Laments

It's my birthday, and I'll cry if I want to. I feel awful, am weepier than usual, and have to address cancer on a daily basis. I wanted to ignore the day. I didn't want to have anything, do anything, or treat the day as anything more than a typical day. No cake! But my girls called several times during the week. I received phone and e-mail birthday greetings from my sisters and cards from well-wishers. Matt sent a beautiful rose bouquet to my school. So now my colleagues are wishing me well and I'm a puddle of tears. I decided that I owed myself a birthday gift. Screw being an obedient do-bee! I canceled radiation, picked up Petie, and drove to the beach to walk along the shore. In the fall, the beaches here are wide, empty, and just beautiful. Petie and I took a long walk. We came home to Matt getting ready to cook up fabulous home-grown tomatoes stuffed with lobster salad and champagne. Have I mentioned what a good man I have? Champagne, in the middle of the week, is such a great idea—better than cake. November 9 is still my very last day of treatment, no matter what!

Thanks for listening. You are all such a blessing.
Hug everyone you know.
Antoinette

From: Anne St. John
To: Antoinette
Date: Friday, October 19, 2007 at 4:00 p.m.
Subject: Birthday Laments

Welcome to the club! I was waiting for what celebration was scheduled, but I see you're keeping it quiet. That doesn't mean I can't take you out! How about next Saturday? We could go Chinese or Italian. Is Friday better?

Anne

~

From: Pam B
To: Antoinette
Date: Friday, October 19, 2007 at 4:52 p.m.
Subject: Birthday Laments

Oh Ann, sooooooooooooo sorry I blew your big day! But it sounds like forgetting all about it was just what you wanted. Why did you think you were going to sail right through this cancer thing without getting grumpy and weepy?! No one else expected you to. You and Pam have the same "I'm ignoring that I have cancer" thing going on, but I think you are only making it harder on yourself! And you know, it's sad that your bust-out radical move is a walk on the beach with Petie! I hope you are up to some adoration because we do our cooking night next weekend and are likely to at least toast you. There may be cake! Love you lots.

Pam B.

~

From: Lisa
To: Antoinette
Date: Saturday, October 20, 2007 at 7:14 a.m.
Subject: Birthday Laments

I understand! I turned forty last April. I was supposed to have chemo that day but delayed a day because I just didn't want that as a gift. Regardless, it was a tough chemo phase. I was completely bald, and my eyelashes and eyebrows had just gone. I was also a strange color. I told Rob I wanted to cancel my birthday. I would do forty, but not until I had two breasts and eyebrows.

Well, that time has come. I am going to have a party to celebrate my redo—November 10. I would be thrilled if you and Matt would come (but understand if you aren't up for it). It is also nearly my one-year anniversary. Lots to celebrate and be thankful for. You are a warrior, and you are winning.

XXOO -L

~

From: Dr. Pam
To: Antoinette
Date: Monday, October 22, 2007 at 6:55 a.m.
Subject: Birthday Laments

I thought of you on the 18th. Think of fifty as another milestone. And don't sweat missing a radiation session now and then. They are zapping you with enough to do the job. The chemo crap we went through this summer killed any cancer cells that were floating around. Remember the radiation is only to prevent the REMOTE chance of local recurrence. My mastectomy is your radiation. You are very patient. I knew I never could go every day and be reminded. This whole cancer thing pisses me off. I have no eyebrows or eyelashes now. A small bit of fuzz on my head. Stay strong. Looking forward to fifty more years together walking on the beach.

Pam

Aunt Kay and Uncle Phil's anniversary party was fabulous. My aunt looked stunning in her golden gown, and Uncle Phil was dressed so handsomely in his tuxedo. They both smiled bright and proud all night. The food was fabulous and the band so much fun, as was catching up with my cousins, aunts, and uncles. I was heartened to see Diana and Barbara talking, hugging, and happy to be in each other's company. My dress fit well, and I felt good, healthy, and very happy to be in a room full of people I loved so dearly. At the end of the night, Matt and I danced to a slow song. He pulled me close and dropped his head into my neck.

"Don't start, baby," I whispered. "We have everything to be happy about."

"I know," he sniffed.

Sometimes my big, strong man proved to be a bigger puddle than me.

chapter forty-seven

Permission

I did go back for treatment the day after my birthday. No one asked why I had missed the previous day's appointment, so I did not volunteer an excuse.

The following Monday, I lay strapped and elevated on the table with the gun pointed at the just-right spot when, suddenly, drips of liquid fell on my neck and shoulder. I was quickly taken down and had to sit in the waiting room while they assessed the situation.

Finally, the technician explained that the machine was down. "We will call you if it is not fixed by your appointment tomorrow," he said.

"Does this session count?"

"No, you will have to make up this one up."

I shook my head as I got up to go the dressing room. "No," I said, "I plan to be absolutely done on November 9."

The machine was up and running the next day. After the session, the nurse lumbered in as I was being released from the straps.

"You do realize you have to make up the sessions you missed," she said.

This woman was just as sullen as most of the staff I had met there. She loomed over me, tall and demanding.

I took a breath. "We'll see," I said as I sidestepped around her to leave the room.

"Unbelievable!" she exclaimed to the technicians as I left. I was sure she meant for me hear.

I drove to my parents' house. We were officially moving in a few days, and I had boxes to bring over. Mom was preparing dinner. While she chopped celery, I complained about the cold doctor, the sour nurse, and the surly technician. I cried through several napkins. Mom had not encountered anyone like that while going through her treatments. She said everyone had been kind, respectful, and caring.

"This is not a nice place, Antoinette," she said, handing me a glass of wine.

"I wonder if I could go back to Sloan to finish this," I mused.

Mom took the lid off the bubbling pot. "You could call and find out." She stirred the chicken soup. "You know, I didn't finish the radiation," she said, looking into the pot as she stirred. "I missed a few sessions here and there. We had plane tickets to go away."

"How many did you miss?"

"Three or maybe four. It was fine. They gave me plenty. And I was so tired. I needed a vacation, and so did Daddy."

I took a long sip of wine. My mother always followed the rules. She carefully measured ingredients called for in her recipes, tracked the protocols to the tiniest detail for her lab experiments, made sure the mobile mammography van requirements and paperwork were up to date and satisfactory, no matter how trivial. She was the one who reminded me to listen to the doctors, do what I was told. There were reasons for the procedures. If I followed the rules, I would be all right. I would be safe. Now she was telling me she had taken a shortcut because, at the time, she needed to.

I put down my glass and hugged my mother. I bent over her, wrapped my arms completely around to give her a long, hard hug, the kind I savor from my girls, thinking, *I should do this more often.* "Thanks, Mommy."

~

From: Antoinette
To: Sherry and Janet
Date: Tuesday, October 23, 2007 at 7:45 p.m.
Subject: Radiation Laments

Hi, Sherry and Janet. Being that you two have gone through what I am now going through, I was hoping you could help me with a few questions about the radiation. I believe I made a BIG mistake going to a nearby radiation facility rather than staying with Memorial Sloan Kettering for the sake of convenience. How many sessions did you go through? I was originally quoted at 25–28 total at Sloan; 33 at Riverhead, with the only reason offered for the discrepancy being "that's the way we do it here." This was by far a lame justification, especially when it came from the doctor. Can you imagine what would happen to our careers if we used that line with the families we work with? I am also finding the techs, doc, and nurse communicate badly between each other. I see the doc once a week for a skin check; a day or so later the nurse comes into the radiation room while I'm up high on the table to order blood work. The next day, the princess tech with an attitude that my kids would get a smack in the back of the head for tells me I need blood work. When I told her I had gone the day before, she says no one let her know. It takes three to four days to get results back to their office. It is my fault for not researching better, but I'm just so fed up. I have little confidence in the advice, especially when I am blown off most of the time. For a ten-minute procedure, you would think they could, at least, be considerate and cordial rather than give me the impression that I am imposing on their time (they must have to wait for me since there is usually no one waiting when I arrive). Although chemo at Sloan was scary, the staff was always wonderful, always answered my stupidest questions even when I asked more than once. I always felt they were in the business of getting me through everything with respect and kindness. I get the feeling that this place is simply doing business. Am I being too overly sensitive? Should I just put up with the rudeness? I have thirteen sessions to go. I wish I could finish up at Sloan. Thanks for letting me rant.

Hug everyone you know.
Toni

~

From: Sherry
To: Antoinette
Date: Tuesday, October 23, 2007 at 9:18 p.m.
Subject: Radiation Laments

Stony Brook was great for radiation. I had thirty treatments. They called in advance if the machine was broken (two or three times, so I didn't have to make the trip). The nurse suggested the aloe cream up front, and I was able to avoid more serious side effects. I saw the doctor weekly, and he was part of a team that had Friday morning breakfast meetings to discuss treatments of current patients. The techs were supportive and respectful to me 100 percent of the time, and I seldom had a female tech! There were also other patients in the waiting area going through the same thing, so I knew I wasn't alone! I knew about blood work in advance, and I only had to inquire about results once.

I'm not sure what would be involved with a change, so I'm not sure if it's worth switching at this point. Fill out post-treatment questionnaires and be brutally honest. Maybe you could mention your concerns to a supervising nurse or MD. You are almost done! Hugs and love,

Sherry

From: Janet
To: Antoinette
Date: Thursday, October 25, 2007 at 3:31 p.m.
Subject: Radiation Laments

Damn those BITCHES!!! Write a scathing letter and send it. In the meantime, get it done. I don't think you would be able to switch. Those bitches are obviously not getting any good-bye cookies. Let me know how it goes.

Janet

~

From: Antoinette
To: Sherry and Janet
Date: Thursday, October 25, 2007 at 4:29 p.m.
Subject: Radiation Laments

I talked with my oncology nurse at Memorial Sloan Kettering today. She was sorry to hear about the troubles, but the logistics to switch are not worth it, and I may not get covered by insurance. I have to buck up. I will, however, write a lengthy and honest review when I'm done, and I will not have any follow-up there. November 9 it is. I am not making up any sessions. Thank you for letting me vent. Thank you for your kindness, your friendship, and great suggestions.

Hug everyone you know.
Toni

chapter forty-eight

My Old Pink Room

Nick came over to help Matt move our bed out of the Remsenburg house, into the truck, and up the stairs in my parents' house into my old pink room. It was still pink. Willow perched herself on top of our bed as soon as I put the familiar comforter on top. Matt hooked up a portable TV to the creative cable lines my dad had weaved in and out of rooms throughout the house. I set up my computer in my sisters' old yellow room, where twin beds waited for Hallie and Robyn to visit. Petie was now officially installed at Helga's, along with his dishes, harness, sweater, and bed.

My old pink room was neither big nor small. There was a dresser along one wall; a closet took up half the opposite wall. The bed fit along the north side, giving us a spectacular view through the large wall window looking over the backyard and Great South Bay—the view I grew up with. I anticipated witnessing angry waves crashing into the bulkhead, watching the moon drift across serene nights, and waking up to eastern skies stained in red and purple. With some careful organization, Matt and I could fit in my childhood room. The beauty of the scenes was worth the tight squeeze.

My parents welcomed us into their house, complete with the Rubbermaid containers we cluttered the basement with and our ongoing projects, anxieties, and quirks. Our schedules coincided closely enough that we didn't disturb their routines. Dad had grown up in a crowded multi-generation home. He liked everyone to be in close proximity of each other. There was a comfort in numbers, in always being in the company of love. But this was the first time in my adult life I had found myself and my stuff back in this house, with my parents, in my old pink room.

Mom was up soon after dawn, toasting bread and pouring coffee. Dad liked the televisions and/or a static-y radio on in every room—on high volume, since both he and Mom were steadily losing their hearing. The conservative ranting from their news shows filled the whole house. Matt and I had no desire to listen to the blaring rhetoric. I felt guarded in having to explain moods, preferences in foods, political and environmental opinions, and volume settings. I knew that my private self would not only be in full view of my parents but also my sisters and brother and their families, who frequently dropped by.

Still, my parents were doing us a huge favor in letting us stay with them. We would be close to the building site and save money. I also knew that since I was taking too long to shake off the treatments' exhausting side effects, having Mom in the kitchen and willing to pick up anything at the grocery store would give me much-needed breaks. I prepared myself for feelings of guilt over the complaints that would inevitably crop up. I resigned myself to the fact that my old pink room—the tightly packed 9x12 space that overlooked the temperaments of the Great South Bay—would be my sanctuary for the next six months or so.

chapter forty-nine

Moving On

I placed a bucket of candy on the front porch of the Remsenburg house during my lunch break on Halloween day. Although few children lived in the immediate neighborhood and the school PTO hosted a Halloween party during the early evening to keep the young ghouls and fairy princesses off the unlit streets, happily playing on a sugar high, I did not want to chance my almost-sold house becoming a victim of "innocent fun." I thought it prudent to avoid the tricks by offering Tootsie Pops and Baby Ruth candy bars on Halloween Night. If the kids or raccoons did not empty the plastic jack-o-lantern's contents, then Dad and Matt could enjoy the treats on All Saints' Day.

On Sunday morning, I woke weary from all of the physical and emotional punishment of moving, but I had one last trip to the Remsenburg house to make. Matt and I drove out with a toolbox, rakes, and a fresh box of lawn bags bouncing in the back of the truck. I gave the floors, counters, mirrors, and sinks one last wipe-down. Fingerprints were sprayed off the walls. Matt finished clearing out the gardens. He salvaged the last of the tomato cages, collected a batch of oregano, and trimmed down the Montauk daisies.

I remembered that I had buried a plastic statue of Saint Joseph, the patron saint of home, in the herb garden. The legend contended that if the statue was buried upside down in a favored outdoor spot, the house sale would be expedited and profitable. Unfortunately, St. Joe had no power over a falling economy. It had taken two years and substantial price lowering to get this far.

The other part of the legend was that once the house was sold, St. Joseph had to be exhumed and placed in a prominent place in the new home, ensuring joy and prosperity. Since it had taken so long to sell, plan, and move, we had not yet begun to break ground on the new house, *and* cancer had been added to the mix, so I was not about to take any chances. I dug up the statue and washed and wrapped it in a dishtowel. I planned for St. Joseph to watch over our home building phase while standing on the dresser in my old pink room.

While scooping fallen leaves from the pool cover, Matt discovered a generous tear in the material. The cover had endured ten winter seasons; it should have been replaced. The hardware stores were closed, so Matt decided to pull out the spare boat tarp that sat in the rented storage unit.

The storage space was packed like a Jenga tower. I imagined the boxes, small engine accessories, and sewing machine crashing on top of Matt's head. He claimed to remember that he'd tucked the tarp on the side of the threshold. I didn't remember moving it or even seeing it on my last visit to the storage unit. Happily, he came back unscathed and with the tarp within a half hour.

Back at the house, we quickly re-covered the pool. Not ideal, but secure—good enough for the next day's inspection.

Days grew dark quickly in November. I needed to lie down on a soft horizontal surface. Matt walked through the rooms one last time. He discovered the upstairs thermostat blinking, indicating low batteries. For some unknowable reason, I had a fresh pack of AAA batteries in my pocketbook. The dishwasher, oven, and water heater were in working order; the dryer whirled as it should. Matt noted the amount of oil left in the tank. Done. Finally satisfied, we closed the door on this life chapter. I gave the front porch post a long, thankful hug.

Monday, November 5, 2007: Closing Day

Our appointment was in Rocky Point, on the north shore of Long Island, at eleven thirty. I packed copies of the necessary and probably unnecessary papers in a canvas tote. All of the players were prompt and present—lawyers, realtors, notaries, architects, us, and the buyer's father, whose only job was to quietly observe the process. The office was located in an inconspicuous strip mall. The receptionist, who had a bright red lipstick smile and big, bottled blonde hair directed us to go through the lauan doors into the conference room.

We walked into a room that held a long table with a cheap Formica top, worn chairs, a fax machine, a telephone, and one small window with a vinyl shade pulled down over it. The shabbiness seemed out of place for a client who was paying cash for the house and applying for a huge loan to begin renovations. Matt remained cautious.

Paper shuffled smoothly for almost two hours. I felt like I was signing my citizenship away. Finally, the notarized check was passed in front of us, and . . . Crap! The check was made out to the bank lawyer and me. We could have shouted, demanded explanations. Instead, we laughed. We were all drained. We agreed to follow the lawyer to the bank for a new check.

While shaking everyone's hand, the buyer's father asked for the name and phone number of our landscaper. He admired the details of the flower and vegetable gardens throughout the property. I told him Matt and I took care of the gardens ourselves, and we paid a local young man to mow the lawn—a kid who'd showed up at the front door in May after competing in the South Pacific surfing circuit.

I made it back to the radiation facility in time for the session.

The belligerent nurse handed me the script for the final blood work. "Be sure to get this done today," she ordered.

I stuffed it into my pocketbook, intending to ignore it. It was not worth a vein stick with just four more sessions to go.

❋

chapter fifty

Standing Firm

When I came in for radiation a few days later, the doctor attempted to have a heart-to-heart talk with me. I was not prepared for a conversation, since we'd never really had one before.

The doctor expressed her bewilderment over my non-compliant attitude and refusal to make up the two sessions I'd missed. I lamely listed my reasons: Work had grown demanding. I had just moved and was exhausted. She retorted that these excuses were not sufficient to jeopardize my health. Confrontation without a rehearsal had never been my strength. I took a breath. I blurted out that I was not convinced that these last two radiation sessions were imperative because she never explained the discrepancy between the Memorial Sloan Kettering's recommendations and hers.

Unbelievably, she went into a detailed dissertation. She outlined how the amount of *rads* and timing of the treatments were calculated. The staging and location of the original tumor and the surgical margins were all taken into consideration. She threw out vaguely familiar physics terms. It sounded impressive, although six weeks too late. She could not convince me that the last two radiation sessions would make the difference between life and death. The sole purpose of radiation therapy was to ensure that cancer never returns to the affected breast—to the one spot on that breast. If cancer should ever reappear, it was not going to be in that breast. I did not argue. I let her ramble on.

With an exasperated sigh, she theorized that perhaps I was not taking her seriously because she looked so young. Really?

It was time to put this ego in its place. I exclaimed how uncomfortable I felt with the negative vibes and discourteous attitudes from the technicians and nurse as well as from her. The curt replies, talking over me as if I did not need to understand, the impatience. They may have the skill set, but basic compassion and kindness were sorely lacking.

The doctor stood up and smoothed her skirt with my file. This conversation had taken too much of her time. She said she was sorry to hear this. I should have mentioned it to her sooner. However, if I did not complete the treatment as prescribed, she would have to report my insubordinations to my oncologist (she was going to tell on me!).

I shrugged and said they were aware of my discontent and my feeling that I'd made a big mistake coming to this facility. The doctor jotted a quick note, looked up, and stated that my last treatment was scheduled for Tuesday, November 13.

As she left the room, the nurse cut in front of my exit. "Didn't you get the blood work done?"

"Nope."

"Here is another script," she said, handing me the paper.

"I won't need it," I said, pulling my robe tighter. "Tomorrow is my last day."

I felt a little shaky lying on the table for that second-to-last hit. Princess Tech was especially dismissive. I did my best to ignore her.

Standing up for myself had taken previously untapped bravery. While driving home to Sayville, a million witty comebacks came to mind. But I did not shed one tear.

part three

Home Stretch

chapter fifty-one

Done! Done! Done!

On November 9, 2007, I walked into the facility at four fifteen, undressed, lay like a limp piece of meat, got zapped, and got down off the table and out the door within fifteen minutes. I confirmed with the receptionist, one of the courteous few, that I would not be in next week nor need a follow-up appointment. I shook her hand and thanked her for her thoughtful attention.

Earlier that day, the kindergarten class had thrown me a surprise "Hurray for Mrs. Martin" party during their afternoon snack. Debbie Johnson explained to the children that I had accomplished a very hard job. They were all proud of me for persevering through the challenges.

"Mrs. Martin showed us strong character traits. She is our role model," Mrs. Johnson said to the children. She had a way of weaving curriculum standards into every minute.

Twenty-two little faces beamed at me. The little girls wore pink dresses and bows. I read my *Famous Seaweed Soup* storybook to them, even though it was out of season. We had fresh vegetables with ranch dressing dip, pretzels shaped as support ribbons, pink-and-white M&Ms, and juice boxes. Each child signed an oversized card. One little boy pulled at my hand to say, "This is like a birthday party, except you are big!"

My heart swelled as I gave this sweet boy a hug of gratitude.

chapter fifty-two

The Letter

November 9, 2007

Dear Doctor,

Since your office does not send out a "How did you like your treatment" questionnaire, I thought I'd write a letter. I tend to be a better writer than talker, and I do not want you to think that I am an oppositional witch. Quite the contrary, I am typically a very good "do-bee," so long as there is respect.

This was the first time I had ever been sick. All of my medical experiences, and my family's, have been thankfully routine and never life-threatening. Through the years, physicians I have had were forthcoming and kind, creating a compatible patient-physician partnership. The tone of their care trickled down to their staff, making the environment comfortable and trusting. I know the value of developing a repertoire, given that this is what my clients and parents of my students desperately look for in professionals who are entrusted with their care and future. In my almost thirty years of professional experience, I have prided myself on making sure everyone is comfortably on the same page.

Cancer has been a very, very scary journey for not only me but also for my husband, children, parents, sisters, brothers, large extended family, and circle of caring friends. It has been an arduous year in keeping myself calm and focused so that everyone else can remain calm as I navigated through.

Through my diagnosis, surgery, and chemotherapy, I have encountered unbelievably patient, knowledgeable doctors, courteous nurses and techs, and caring phone receptionists. Never, ever was I made to feel that my volley of questions and anxieties were unimportant. I did not always like what they had to say and do, but they made sure I understood every option and every step for each option. My whole well-being was truly cared about. Details were addressed, time expended, and a relationship of trust was established on the first consult visit. We could all calm down and plow forward. I was confident to put my life in these professionals' hands.

I believed that this was the standard in the oncology field. The doctors and team of professionals are not only educated and experienced, but they also have to be so understanding, kind, and courteous to be with cancer patients all day long, every day. It must be a very hard job.

When it came time for the grind of the daily radiation treatments, I started a new job and was moving from Remsenburg to Sayville. My doctors at Memorial Sloan Kettering agreed that I should find a more convenient location. This part of the treatment was supposed to be a cakewalk as compared to diagnosis, surgery, and chemotherapy.

After the first consult with you, I was more confused as to the hows and whys of the protocol. When I asked further questions, you just repeated the presentation. I walked out in a daze of uncertainty. After discussing everything with my husband, we decided that all questions would soon be answered, and my anxieties would be put to rest. This was not supposed to be hard! I should have known that first impressions set the tone. It was my mistake not to listen to my initial instincts.

Feelings of uncertainty were compounded by the nurse and some of the techs' rude attitudes. The eye rolling and sighing were especially unnerving, making the daily visits even more uncomfortable. I got the feeling that I was putting everyone out.

When I asked again about the protocol during the first examination after treatment started, your reply, with your hand on the doorknob, was, "That's the way we do things here." I was officially blown off! It became very clear that your only concern for me was the condition of the skin on the right breast. I should blindly follow what you say. You did not ask anything. You gave a cursory greeting. You were obviously not listening anyway. There was no way I could comfortably come to you with any issues!

At one point, I called my oncologist to see if there was a way for me to continue at Memorial Sloan Kettering. I no longer cared about time and traffic. The radiation oncologist was not comfortable because I was already mapped and in the middle of treatment. My oncologist and nurse actively listened and sympathized but encouraged me to just finish. I was stuck. All I could do was remain quiet and set my sights on Day 33—November 9.

When the date neared, the techs realized that I was two sessions short and I was not coming in past November 9. Now you wanted to communicate. I must admit your justification for thirty-three sessions vs. twenty-seven was very good—six weeks too late, but good. It is obvious that you are a very bright and ambitious doctor. Even so, I am not convinced that the two missed sessions put me at any more of a risk. I am sure the radiation I did receive was more than enough. I am exhausted from the anxiety of walking into that office each day. I am done. I will not be back. You can put that on my permanent record.

For that record, your appearance did not play into my first impressions. You are indeed blessed with youthful looks, but I did the math. You have to be in your forties to be in the position you are in.

Cancer will always loom over my shoulder. I am lucky in being diagnosed so early. I have an excellent chance for survival. I have full confidence in my Memorial Sloan Kettering oncologists and know they will see me through whatever has to be done to stay well and keep cancer at bay. Through this last leg of the journey, I learned that I will now pay very close attention to my initial impressions and never, ever weigh convenience over a sure thing. Perhaps you may take heed and pay attention to how you and your staff communicate with each other and with your patients. We tend to be a bit more complicated than skin burns.

Sincerely,
Antoinette T. Martin

I not only wrote the letter, I actually mailed it! It felt great to have a final say. A few weeks later, the facility's office manager called to ask if I would send her a copy of the letter. She had heard about it but had not been able to read it. I told her I had mailed it directly to the doctor and had no intention of pursuing issues any further. She assured me that I would not be involved and that the letter would be used for professional development purposes. I printed and mailed her a copy. Perhaps some good would come of it.[1]

From: Antoinette
To: My Everyone
Date: Friday, November 9, 2007 at 8:43 p.m.
Subject: ALL DONE!

We had a week of met milestones. Last weekend Matt and I officially cleared out our Remsenburg house. I remembered to dig up the St. Joseph's statue from the herb garden because I was not going to mess with any "juju." We discovered a major tear in the pool cover that should have been replaced a season or two before. Matt took his life in his hands and pulled the extra boat cover from storage. Our Remsenburg house was such a good home for us. We will easily forget our frustrations but always love the memories.

Closing day went surprisingly smooth. Two hours of paper shuffling and signing.

Matt and I are now living at my parents' house. We are in my old bedroom; it is still pink! The sunrise over the bay is spectacular from my window. Petie is in foster care with Matt's mom and sister. Willow came with us and shares the

---

1 Almost a year after I sent that letter, I ran into a technician at the local CVS. She occasionally substituted for the regular techs and was one of the few with a kind word and sincere compassion. She stopped me in the cough and cold aisle to thank me for writing that letter, saying, "Concerns were addressed, and some good changes are happening."

pink room. My parents are easy to live with. However, the other night when Matt drove upstate to see Robyn's art exhibit and I went to the city with friends for a celebration, Dad fell into his dad role asking who was driving (the train), who was I with (my best buds, the Bensons) and when would I be home (?). My two-minute commute to work was increased to 25 minutes. But it's a smooth ride going the opposite way of traffic—a decompression commute. Presently, we are wrestling with town permits and still talking with builders. It should be coming together soon.

But the best closing ever is that I am officially all done with cancer treatment! YAHOO!!! What a relief. My kindergarten class surprised me on Friday afternoon with a "Hooray for Mrs. Martin" party! Precious.

Cancer will always loom over me. I have complete trust in my MSKCC oncologist to help me keep this beast at bay. In the meantime, there is so much of life to live! What an incredible blessing to have all of you beside me, encouraging me and keeping an ear open.

The holidays are coming up. I'll be strangling my girls with hugs soon. My good man beside me, fun friends and family nearby, football on Sundays, a good night's sleep—all good things to be thankful for. Every day is a gift.

Hug everyone you know.
Antoinette

From: Mary
To: Antoinette
Date: Saturday, November 10, 2007 at 8:22 a.m.
Subject: ALL DONE!

Excellent—only look forward, never back. Love you,

Mary

~

From: Colleen
To: Antoinette
Date: Saturday, November 10, 2007 at 10:18 a.m.
Subject: ALL DONE!

You did it, girlfriend! I am so proud of you. When and where is the celebration?

Colleen XXOO

~

The burns around my breast and up my chest to the base of my neck were very raw. Fatigue wrapped through every inch of my body, weighing down attempts to move. The mind fog still muddled my thoughts and memory. But this would be as bad as it could possibly get. From now on, I was on the mend in both mind and body.

❊

epilogue

October 2014

A low ceiling of gray clouds hung over the bayside beach. A brisk northwest wind blew short waves onto the shallows. Just two hundred yards offshore, the bay would be wild and cold.

Matt and I had rented an oceanfront beach house for the entire summer season. He commuted to the mainland on most workdays; I soaked in much-needed Vitamin D, ocean swims, beach walks, writing, and sailing. But now the days had shortened and temperatures had cooled. Summer was over. Our little fleet of boats needed to be pulled from the bay and tucked in for winter's hibernation. This was the last weekend I could sail my Sunfish to the mainland.

I wore a long-sleeve T-shirt under a life jacket and sailing gloves. There was a wicked wind to sail me five miles across the bay in record time. Matt shoved me off, promising to catch up in the motorboat, which had recently been plagued with a number of engine ailments. He was on his own.

Within minutes, the waves crashed across the bow and the hull heeled at a precarious angle. I carefully released and pulled back the mainsheet, controlling the sail to steady the course. I aimed to get across in one tack. My feet held onto the cockpit straps, my heft, leaning windward, struggled to balance. I held the tiller to steer up breaking crests and crash down to the valleys. I knew I would be sporting a bloom of bruises as a testimony to these bumps and slaps. It was worth it.

The hull hummed. The wind howled. I howled back. Here I soared, a fifty-seven-year-old woman with Stage IV breast cancer, screaming into the wind, "You can't catch me!"

December 2014

It took me seven years to write this memoir. I saved the reams of e-mails and that ugly journal I kept during that year of cancer just so I could tell the story. I thought it would be clever to add the e-mails in the diary format. I schemed that my journey could be easily told with humor and lighthearted quips. But each time I attempted to execute my plan, anxiety paralyzed me, providing excuses to put the writing away. Cancer was not a whimsical journey. Perhaps it should never be told. I never wanted to face it again.

In 2012, however, cancer did return, as it does for more than 30 percent of early-stage breast cancer patients. Somehow, tenacious little cells survived the systemic chemotherapy and bypassed breast tissue and the nodes to settle and grow on my lower vertebrae. I am now living with Stage IV breast cancer that metastasized to my spine. Presently, I am fine. It was caught early enough, before any real damage occurred. The treatment protocols are not too invasive or interruptive—no ports or infusion sessions. I am still a wimp when it comes to the frequent vein sticks, but my oncology team at Memorial Sloan Kettering Cancer Center remains understanding and accommodating. I continue to work, take care of my family and home, and live my life with the people I cherish.

This new diagnosis gave me permission to do what I had always known I should be doing: write. I enrolled in the Stony Brook/Southampton MFA in Creative Writing and Literature program. It gave me confidence, community, and a voice to tell the stories that have been playing out in my head for far too long. I was back in school and loving everything about it.

Before I could write the stories I wanted to tell, I had to first muster courage and write the story that was hardest. I found the process difficult, scary, and, some days, unwelcoming. Luckily, Memorial Sloan Kettering Cancer Center had a writers' program for patients. I was serendipitously matched up with Robert Sam Anson, a cancer survivor and gifted writer and editor. He encouraged me to start the story and mentored me as I began.

Writing this memoir has shown me that I am a capable, albeit laboring, writer. More revealing was that I was braver than I ever would have thought possible. It was only because I was always neck-deep in blessings and love. Writing this memoir gave me the power to know that I can navigate through this new cancer. Perhaps my story can give others a means to find their strength and hope.

I do not plan on a sequel. I decided that while I can, I will keep this new cancer on a carefully watched low burner. It does not deserve my full attention or a journal dedicated to its presence. I refuse to give it voice or call it mine. I have too much life on my plate, too many stories to write.

acknowledgments

No one accomplishes a feat like writing a book without a tribe of believers and supporters. I owe a sincere thank-you to so many.

Heartfelt thanks to Brooke Warner, publisher of She Writes Press; Lauren Wise, project editor; and the hard-working SWP staff behind the scenes. Their expertise and resolve shepherded this story into a beautiful book.

Daily gratitude goes out to the dedicated Memorial Sloan Kettering Cancer Center oncologists, nurses, technicians, researchers, receptionists, greeters, volunteers . . . everyone. They are the best in the business, and I am living proof. The MSKCC writers' program, Visible Ink, provided the encouragement that made this book possible. Former MSKCC patients volunteer to mentor a current patient's writing project. Robert Sam Anson, a talented writer and editor in his own right, was my mentor and urged me to write my story.

I am so lucky to live nearby and be accepted into the Stony Brook/Southampton MFA Creative Writing and Literature Program. I reveled in each class and sharpened the skills and confidence I needed to write. The faculty and advisors were phenomenal. Special applause goes to Lou Ann Walker, a masterful writer and caring mentor, and Andrew Botsford, a critical reader and editor.

While studying for my MFA, I met two women who soon became my writing buddies. Jackie Goodwin and Melinda

Ferguson repeatedly offered their ears, thoughts, time, and incredible writing skills as I wrought the manuscript into existence. We continue to commiserate over our writing lives, share our art, and encourage each other's projects forward. Their friendship has been invaluable.

Then, there is My Everyone—too numerous to name, but you know who you are. Hugs, kisses, and thanks cannot begin to aknowledge the love I have for all of you in my life. I do want to extend special thanks to my dear friend Colleen Hofmeister, an incredibly brave role model, as we live well past our expiration dates with Stage IV breast cancer. My daughters, Sara, Hallie, and Robyn, deserve public accolades. These young women not only bring my life joy but also humor my big ideas and inspire daily pride that fills my heart. Diana and Bill Truglio—the best parents anyone could ever wish for—must be honored here for providing my foundations of family love and so much more that make life a beautiful journey.

Last and never least, there is my husband and best friend, Matt—the good man. He recognized my need to write and gave me the space I needed to make the ride to publication happen. Strap in, baby; there's more to come.

About the Author

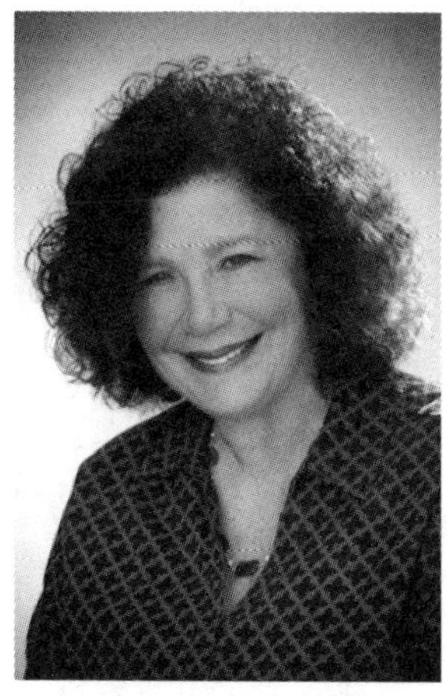

ANTOINETTE TRUGLIO MARTIN is a speech therapist and special education teacher by training but is a writer at heart. She is the author of *Famous Seaweed Soup*, and was a visiting author in schools for several years. She was formerly a regular columnist for *Parent Connection (In A Family Way)* and *Fire Island Tide (Beach Bumming)*. Personal experience essays and excerpts of her memoir have been published in *Bridges (2014)*, *Visible Ink (2015)*, and *The Southampton Review (2016)*. Martin proudly received her MFA in creative writing and literature from Stony Brook Southampton University (2016). As a Stage IV breast cancer patient, she does not allow cancer to dictate her life. She lives in her hometown of Sayville with her husband, Matt, and is never far from My Everyone and the beaches she loves.

SELECTED TITLES FROM SHE WRITES PRESS

She Writes Press is an independent publishing company founded to serve women writers everywhere. Visit us at www.shewritespress.com.

The Longest Mile: A Doctor, a Food Fight, and the Footrace that Rallied a Community Against Cancer by Christine Meyer, MD. $16.95, 978-1-63152-043-3. In a moment of desperation, after seeing too many patients and loved ones battle cancer, a doctor starts running team—never dreaming what a positive impact it will have on her community.

Beautiful Affliction: A Memoir by Lene Fogelberg. $16.95, 978-1-63152-985-6. The true story of a young woman's struggle to raise a family while her body slowly deteriorates as the result of an undetected fatal heart disease.

Body 2.0: Finding My Edge Through Loss and Mastectomy by Krista Hammerbacher Haapala. An authentic, inspiring guide to reframing adversity that provides a new perspective on preventative mastectomy, told through the lens of the author's personal experience.

Renewable: One Woman's Search for Simplicity, Faithfulness, and Hope by Eileen Flanagan. $16.95, 978-1-63152-968-9. At age forty-nine, Eileen Flanagan had an aching feeling that she wasn't living up to her youthful ideals or potential, so she started trying to change the world—and in doing so, she found the courage to change her life.

Don't Leave Yet: How My Mother's Alzheimer's Opened My Heart by Constance Hanstedt. $16.95, 978-1-63152-952-8. The chronicle of Hanstedt's journey toward independence, self-assurance, and connectedness as she cares for her mother, who is rapidly losing her own identity to the early stage of Alzheimer's.

Warrior Mother: A Memoir of Fierce Love, Unbearable Loss, and Rituals that Heal by Sheila K. Collins, PhD. $16.95, 978-1-938314-46-9. The story of the lengths one mother goes to when two of her three adult children are diagnosed with potentially terminal diseases.